HOW TO AGE-PROOF YOUR DOG

HOW TO AGE-PROOF YOUR DOG

The Art and Science of Successful Canine Aging

Elizabeth U. Murphy

ROWMAN & LITTLEFIELD
Lanham • Boulder • New York • London

Published by Rowman & Littlefield
A wholly owned subsidary of The Rowman & Littlefield Publishing Group,
Inc.
4501 Forbes Boulevard, Suite 200, Lanham, Maryland 20706
www.rowman.com

Unit A, Whitacre Mews, 26-34 Stannary Street, London SE11 4AB

British Library Cataloguing in Publication Information Available

Library of Congress Cataloging-in-Publication Data

Names: Murphy, Elizabeth U., 1958- , author.
Title: How to age-proof your dog : the art and science of successful canine aging / Elizabeth U.
    Murphy.
Description: Lanham : Rowman & Littlefield, 2017. | Includes bibliographical references and
    index.
Identifiers: LCCN 2016035120 (print) | LCCN 2016053901 (ebook) | ISBN 9781442247161
    (cloth : alk. paper) | ISBN 9781442247178 (Electronic)
Subjects: LCSH: Dogs. | Dogs--Aging. | Dogs--Health. | Veterinary geriatrics.
Classification: LCC SF427 .M97 2017 (print) | LCC SF427 (ebook) | DDC 636.7--dc23
LC record available at https://lccn.loc.gov/2016035120

∞ ™ The paper used in this publication meets the minimum requirements of
American National Standard for Information Sciences—Permanence of Paper
for Printed Library Materials, ANSI/NISO Z39.48-1992.

Printed in the United States of America

To Mark—best husband, best friend.

CONTENTS

I

AGE-PROOFING?

The afternoon knows what the morning never suspected. —Robert Frost

In the United States during the second decade of the twenty-first century, we are, by popular reputation, a youth-obsessed society. However, despite the abundance of magazine covers, TV shows, and movies full of slender, athletic, and attractive twentysomethings, numerous advertisements and infomercials are also full of tips to prevent the aging process. Therefore, our society is really more of an *age*-obsessed society. We are *all* getting older at the same rate, and, as we watch our parents age, many of us are worrying about our own aging process, and some of us seek ways to prevent it.

The thing is—we can't. Aging is inevitable. However, aging is *not* a disease—it is really more of a compromise. Associated with aging are changes we can't avoid, and some we just have to learn to live with. But, since some changes associated with aging *are* predictable, we can take steps early in life that modify the degree to which those changes affect how well we live in old age. The fundamental point here is the word "well"—we may or may not be able to take steps to affect how *long* we live, but we all want to age *well*—in the best health possible, in comfort, in dignity, in joy—and the steps to aging *well* start while we are young. Good nutrition, exercise, early and anticipatory care of medical problems—all starting early in life—can make the difference between disability and ability later in life.

How does this relate to our dogs? Well, they are aging right along with us, but faster, much faster. All of us who have owned dogs have felt the same regret as Agnes Sligh Turnbull, who said: "Dogs' lives are too short. Their only fault, really." Again, we can't prevent the aging process in our dogs, and we can't avoid the inevitable result of aging, but we *can* modify the process, and we can change our dogs' pathway to old age starting when we bring them home as puppies.

This book will help you help your dog age successfully. It will provide information that you can use to predict which health problems might occur in your dog so that you can be proactive about them, and so that, teamed with your veterinarian, you can possibly prevent some of them. It will relate some of the aging changes you will inevitably see in your dog with those that occur in humans, and allow you to recognize how it might feel to *be* an aging dog. As I have said before, we humans can be age-obsessed—dogs are not. We humans think, and talk, a lot about aging and how it feels, and we add lots of intellectual and emotional pieces to the mix. I believe that dogs simply feel the way they feel at the time that they feel it, and do not add much more to it than that. Dogs do not seek to understand the aging process, and do not worry about its limitations—they just focus on what they *can* do, not on what they *can't* do, and just keep on doing it.

For example, I recently saw a sixteen-and-half-year-old dog, named Nikki, who still goes jogging with her owners! Many owners wouldn't even think of taking a dog that age for walks, much less runs, because they would assume that an old dog would rather stay home sleeping. Lots of owners focus on their dog's chronology—that is, the age in years, not their dog's ability. Nikki is blind in one eye, but can still see well with the other, can still hear, is slender, muscular, and has some mobility issues, but none of these things interfere with her desire to fetch a ball—so her owners keep throwing it! She gets up every single morning with a purpose—she has been chasing the cat in the house, Baxter, every morning for the past ten years—she apparently looks forward to it (she starts whining to get out of the bedroom at 6 a.m.). Baxter also apparently looks forward to it (he waits in the hallway in the morning, occasionally sticking his paw under the bedroom door). The owners (when they aren't trying to sleep late) apparently appreciate the show. After all, everybody needs a job, and this dog has one (and so does Baxter, by the way). Nikki does what she can do, which is a *lot*, and definitely does not think at all about what she can't do, and, luckily, neither do her owners.

This book will help you, the dog owner, think like a dog, but act, on your dog's behalf, like a human, allowing your dog's older years to be as comfortable and positive as possible. I want to emphasize that the goal is *not* simply to extend your dog's lifespan, although the information and tips presented may help do so—the goal is actually to help you extend your dog's "healthspan." This is a term used in aging research to distinguish between "lifespan," the period between birth and death, and "healthspan," the period during which a person or animal is fully fit and free of serious illness. A chronologically long lifespan may include some time when the quality of life is not very good, whereas a long healthspan should include less or none of that time—and, of course, we all want the best quality of life possible for our dogs for as long as possible. To paraphrase the Irish serenity prayer, my purpose in writing this book is to grant dog owners the serenity to accept the things they cannot change; the courage to change the things they can; and the wisdom to know the difference.

And who am I to tell anyone anything about this? I am a small-animal veterinarian who has been in practice, in the *same* practice, for eighteen years. The same dogs and cats that I saw as puppies and kittens in my first year of practice have now gone through their geriatric years, and I have seen them through all of their wellness visits as well as all of their illnesses. Some have passed away now, and, after grieving alongside their owners, I have been entrusted in the care of another generation of puppies. Seeing the trajectory of the lives of these dogs, along with those of their owners', has allowed me to understand my ability to affect both.

I have, perhaps, a different perspective on this matter than some other veterinarians—I was, before attending the Cornell College of Veterinary Medicine, a physician assistant, and have had a tendency to view the practice of veterinary medicine from a human medicine perspective. The practice of human medicine, as taught to me at Duke University's Physician Assistant Program, had a more holistic approach than some aspects of veterinary medicine has traditionally had—that is, the practitioner should take into account all of the factors that affect the patient's health, including the emotional and social pieces related to their lives outside the exam room. Being the veterinarian who has been privileged to take care of these dogs and cats all these years has involved more than just keeping track of their required vaccines, heartworm tests, and parasite checks—it has included getting to know their owners and watching them enjoy, and occasionally struggle with, puppyhood, then adulthood, and then the senior years. I have watched how these dogs, as they change, have had an impact on their owners' lives, and how their owners have adapted their lifestyles and their homes to compensate for the aging changes in their dogs. I have watched the owners' lives change, too, and have seen how *that* impacts the place their dogs have in their lives. I, too, am aging, and have seen my parents age as well. This combination of professional and life experiences has made me think, perhaps in a unique way, about the way that some of the techniques that humans use to improve the process of aging in humans could be adapted for use by the caretakers of dogs to help their dogs age well.

In humans, knowledge about the aging process is expanding every day (in part, because our dogs are being used as a model of human aging) and strategies to help compensate for aging changes start with the knowledge of what we humans have to begin with, and how those things change as time goes on. To help our dogs age well, we must first understand the physical and mental abilities they have; it is only with that knowledge that we can first preserve them for as long as possible, and then compensate for them as they change.

This book will train you to be your dog's life coach, personal trainer, and occupational therapist by giving you the knowledge and tools to be an ongoing barometer of your dog's state of health—both physical and mental—to promote the best health possible in your dog, for as long as possible. As you read, you will encounter a lot of science. You may think you hate science and you may be tempted to skip through some of it—if so, that's OK (you can always go back and read it later). But the science presented here will give you a way to understand how and why to age-proof your dog—that's the "art" part in this book's subtitle. That dog with whom you chose to share your life is a complex creature who is the culmination of eons of canine evolution, which you can't actually alter. However, the pathway of your dog's life from now to old age is now in your hands. Which route you choose, and how you steer along the way is totally up to you—you'll encounter some road hazards, but how you maneuver around them will give your dog the best chance to arrive safely at the destination—a healthy old age. After all: "Properly trained, a man can be dog's best friend"—Corey Ford, American writer.

As you read this book, you will notice a few things about how it is written. First, I change the pronoun I use when I refer to dogs—since some readers have male dogs and some have females, I alternate genders from chapter to chapter. Second, I refer to the dogs I treat in the clinic as "patients" while I refer to their owners as "clients." And this brings up the third point—most of the time, I refer to the people that have dogs as "owners"—this seems to push buttons with some "pet parents" and "pet companions," but these terms are a little cumbersome to use, so I chose not to use them. Plus, we really do, legally, own our dogs, even though most of us, and our dogs, know that they own us! One last thing—although you will learn a ton of new things about the health, the personality, and the aging process of your dog (and, perhaps, yourself), new information emerges every day. You will find updated information as it comes out on these topics, as well as greater coverage of some of the material in this book, on the website howtoageproofyour-dog.com. Remember that, although knowledge is power, information is the strength behind that power. My job is to give you strength, so that you can have the power to help your dog live well.

2

WHY DO PEOPLE GET DOGS, ANYWAY?

Dogs are not our whole life, but they make our lives whole.
—Roger Caras

When I was in veterinary school, I came across a curious (to me) concept: when my veterinary professors decided on a course of treatment for an animal, part of that decision was based on whether that animal was a pet, an indoor or outdoor pet, a source of income, or a source of food. The treatment chosen often depended, sometimes unfortunately, on the monetary worth of the animal, not on its worth as a living creature. The price of milk sometimes determined the fate of a sick dairy cow or her calf, and a coughing beagle, kept outdoors as part of a pack of raccoon hunters, did not always get the costly (relative to the owner's income) medication needed to get through a bout of pneumonia. Now, this seemed strange to me because my family had always considered pets to be family members—they lived inside with us, sometimes shared our bedrooms, if not our beds—and we took care of them as absolutely and completely as my parents took care of me.

Dogs and cats have had changing roles recently in the lives of many people, especially in this country. However, consideration of the role of a dog in the life of the owner is still a relevant factor in deciding a lifelong course of preventative health care for that dog. For some of us, dogs are our running buddies, for others, our quiet reading buddies at home. Some have puppies as their trial children before the real ones come along, others have dogs as their empty-nest or retirement companions. Sometimes, people intend their dogs for one role and the dog eventually takes on a new, unforeseen one.

Take Lucy, for example—an English Setter who was purchased by a bachelor, Bob, to hunt birds, and, if she was good at it, to produce more good hunting dogs. She was meant to live outside, but moved inside in very short order, then inhabited the couch, the bed, and basically, anything she wanted. Lucy was the focus of Bob's life—and then Allison came along. Luckily, Allison loved Lucy as much as Bob did. Lucy was their practice child after they got married, until three of the human ones came into their world, but she remained as important a member of Bob's family as all the humans. She was indeed a great hunting dog and was bred, as intended. When delivery time came, Lucy had one large puppy, out of the three in her litter, which got stuck in the birth canal, requiring a C-section. I will never forget the moment when I had to tell Bob this news—he looked at me with a pale face and said, as two enormous tears trickled down his cheeks: "Whatever you do, just save Lucy." We did, but lost two out of the three puppies. Due to the dedicated efforts of our veterinary technicians, who would not give up on that last puppy, little Kate became family member number seven in Bob's family. Lucy is now seventeen years old and still goes bird hunting every fall, although her hunting stints are very brief now. She has had surgery twice for cancer and has been seen twice yearly for eleven years by the veterinary oncologists at nearby Purdue University. She has arthritis and has weekly hydrotherapy (exercise on a water treadmill), physical therapy to keep her joints supple and her muscles strong, acupuncture every other week, massage therapy, a variety of medications and supplements to keep her comfortable, and may get stem cell therapy for her arthritis so she can keep doing her favorite thing—bird hunting. I don't think Bob had all this in mind seventeen years ago, but I do know that he is glad that he has had these tools available for Lucy, and that he still has Lucy. So are Allison, their three daughters, and, of course, Kate.

Then there's Mary and Dolly: the children of an older widow, Mary, decided that she needed a companion to ease her depression after the death of her husband. Mary at first was not in favor of this, until she met Dolly, a three-year-old Humane Society resident. Once their eyes locked, Mary fell in love.

For the past ten years, all of us at the clinic have seen Mary and Dolly walking their two miles twice daily, winter and summer, rain and shine, often wearing matching yellow slickers. I didn't know until last year that slender, active, sharp-minded Mary was actually eighty-three years old! For the past ten years, Dolly provided the reason for Mary to get up every day, kept her active, and helped her stay healthy. Mary, in turn, brought Dolly in twice every year for thorough physical exams, bloodwork, vaccines, and also promptly attended to any illnesses or injuries that developed. Despite this excellent care, Dolly developed cancer this past summer at the age of thirteen. Mary did her best to provide her with the proper treatment and pain control, but we all knew, unfortunately, that Dolly would eventually succumb to her illness no matter what we did. The strain of Dolly's illness produced a remarkable change in Mary. She became forgetful, not remembering whether Dolly had eaten or not, or whether she had given Dolly her medicine— she even lost her checkbook, lost her own medications, and forgot to eat. We began having her come by our clinic twice daily so we could entice Dolly to eat, give her the proper medications (we even found Mary's medications among Dolly's), and make sure Mary herself was OK. Mary told me during one of those visits that she never could have imagined how much a dog could come to mean to a person. And to tell you the truth, despite my years of experience, I didn't know, before Dolly and Mary, how much of a lifeline a pet can be to a person.

Dolly passed away in her sleep one night, laying in her favorite spot under Mary's bed after a brief walk on a beautiful day. One of our veterinary technicians came and got Dolly, and we all worried about how Mary would do after that. Much to my surprise, I got a call from Mary about three days after Dolly's death saying that her children were going to take her to look for another dog at the local shelters. Our staff got on the website of the Indianapolis Humane Society, saw a few candidates, made some calls, got some tips from the wonderful staff there, and found Rose—practically a carbon copy of Dolly, just with shorter legs! We had Mary come by the clinic to look at Rose's photo online (since Mary doesn't "do" the Internet), and it was love at first sight—again. A few days later, Mary was seen striding purposefully by our clinic, back in her routine of twice-daily, two-mile walks. She has gained back some weight, has color in her cheeks, and that sharp spark has reappeared in her eyes. She's even started dating—and is very interested in this new phenomenon of dog-friendly restaurants for her out-ings! Rose loves the new man in Mary's life, by the way.

Knowing whether a dog is intended to fulfill the role of a costume accessory in a purse or a chick magnet at the dog park, a playmate for the kids or a hunting dog on the weekends makes a difference in antici-pating and hopefully preventing certain health problems (although, as the previous anecdotes illustrate, one can never fully anticipate the way a dog can come to inhabit one's life). For example, it is important to know whether a large-breed dog with a genetic tendency to have poorly formed hips or elbows is intended for running many miles every week on a hard surface or just playing fetch occasionally in the soft, grassy backyard—I would want all dogs in those high-risk breeds to be screened as puppies for hip dysplasia, but I might be somewhat more insistent about doing it for the dogs destined for an activity that might traumatize those (possibly) poorly formed hips and, therefore, lead to arthritis. Mobility problems in large, older, dogs are often tragically life-limiting if not anticipated and may be avoided. One of my favorite sayings (probably to the annoyance of my clients!) is "Forewarned is forearmed," and that little platitude has come in handy for many dogs over the years. This philosophy worked out well for thirteen-year-old Stella, for example, a beautiful longhaired German Shepherd, whose hips I had to convince the owners to let me evaluate when she was spayed at the age of six months. We found severe hip dysplasia at that early age, long before any symptoms would have been noticed. Because we knew about this problem so early, Stella's owners and I were proac-tive—we were careful about her weight as well as the type of exercise she should do—to avoid too much trauma to her poorly formed hips. We started her on joint-protection supplements, and we x-rayed her hips every year to monitor how much arthritis, if any, she was develop-ing. When she did develop arthritis, she started nonsteroidal anti-in-flammatory drugs, and, when that was not enough to keep her comfort-able and to keep her moving, she had a hip replacement, and her life of chasing squirrels, going for walks, and protecting her family from the evil postal carrier has continued happily and without pain for many, many years—all because of a little education, a lot of caring, and an eye to Stella's future.

Besides discerning the role a dog is intended to play in an owner's life, I also find it important—and fun—to find out why a particular breed, or mixed-breed, was chosen. These things give me insight not only into the personality of the owner, but also some ability to predict how the personality of the dog will fit with the owner's personality. Certain breeds have very strong personality traits, high or low activity levels, and certain quirky habits, and an owner does not always know these things when choosing a certain breed. For example, someone who chooses a Border Collie because the medium size fits in with the size of the urban backyard may not be prepared for that breed's high activity level and desire to herd everything and everybody. For example, I know a Border Collie who gets very little exercise or stimulation from her sedentary urban lifestyle but has found an outlet for her herding instinct by "herding" the ceiling fan around and around—and around—the owner's dining room table! This is clearly annoying to the owner, but perfectly logical to the dog, given this active breed and the original purpose for which it was developed. When I see a new Border Collie puppy for the first time, I try to see how much the new owner knows about that breed and prepare that person for the fact that these wonderful dogs really, really, *really* need a job—whether it be agility trials, Frisbee contests, sheep-herding on the weekends, several days a week at doggie daycare, or just lots and lots of running. If the owner is given this type of information initially, appropriate outlets for that energy may be found early in that dog's life. If not, that owner may ultimately decide that the bored adult Border Collie is too active, too vocal, or too destructive to keep. Behavior problems, some of which are due to personality clashes with the owner, are the number one reason dogs are given up to shelters and then euthanized. To avoid this, I like to perform a bit of preventative behavioral health care as well as preventative physical health care during my exam times.

Why is this important? As the role of dogs has changed in the lives of owners, the role of owners has changed as well. Dogs have morphed into beloved family members for many people, and their "parents" have morphed into their pet children's health advocates. Many of my clients do heavy-duty research on the nutrition in their dog's food, and many come prepared for their wellness visits with a long list of very good questions. The Internet, of course, has somewhat helped with that, but no matter what vehicle is used to get the information, the desire to obtain information is in many owners. That is paired with the desire to find the best medical care possible, and some owners will go to great lengths and distances to obtain it. I have a client who thought nothing about taking his elderly dog to Oregon by car (mind you, I practice in Indiana) to be fitted for a custom orthotic brace to support an overly flexible joint in her front leg—and that road trip was worth it to both of them for her comfort.

Many people now take charge of their own health care, and they want to do the same with the health care of their pets. This, of course, is where their veterinarian comes in. Gone are the days, hopefully, of the authoritarian, all-knowing, never-questioned health-care provider—human or veterinary—and here come the days of the partnership in health care. There is nothing better for a pet than a knowledgeable, motivated, owner/advocate who is in for the long haul—and there is also nothing better for that pet's veterinarian. I love this, personally—my goal is to keep taking care of that dog or cat until a comfortable, old age is reached after a successful life of health. I want to do this by not only taking excellent care of the pet's health, but also by adding to the education and motivation of that owner, for the health and happiness of all parties. You should expect nothing less from your veterinarian. This book is meant to help you, the owner, know what to look for in your dog throughout life so you can be an active and proactive member of your best friend's health-care team, all the way through the long journey from puppyhood to the senior years. Mr. Rogers once said that the beautiful thing about an imagination is that it allows you to consider potential futures and decide which one is the future you want. Now is the time to look at your dog, imagine that dog's future selves and decide which one you want.

The first step in this journey is to think about why you got your dog in the first place—why this breed and why this particular dog. What is it about this individual that appealed to you then and makes that dog special to you now? It helps to think about your own personality, the activities you enjoy, the goals you have for yourself, and the plans you have for your life. Think about how your dog does, or does not, fit in with these things. Your dog, if you play your cards right, will be riding shotgun with you through many years and many changes in your life, and you will be seeing your dog through many changes as well. Knowing what makes this dog special to you, and what the two of you are capable of doing together, helps you structure the lifestyle needed for you to help your dog age successfully. And, when you reach those senior years, remember what those special, unique things were so many years before, so you can keep looking for them, keep finding them, and keep fanning the flames of them even though some aging changes might be dimming their brightness.

Here is a list of questions I want you to ask yourself—write the answers down and then tuck them in a safe place where you can find them in the future—many, many years in the future. In other words, make a "time capsule" for you and your dog. For your dog's time capsule, stash away things like the impossibly tiny collar your dog wore as a puppy, some tattered favorite toys, some pictures, the receipt from the time he ate the TV remote and needed surgery—or whatever is important to you regarding your life with your dog right now. Add the answers to the questions, and then put it away and dig it out again in ten or fifteen years. Or look at it every year, maybe add to it from time to time and then put it away again. In a decade or so, the contents of this time capsule with the answers to these questions will give you some perspective on your dog and your lives together, and will help you see the puppy in your older dog again—maybe even help you see yourself a bit more clearly.

TIME CAPSULE

Why did you get a dog?
Why did you pick this type of dog?
Why did you pick this dog?
What one word would you use to describe your dog?
What is the first thing you think of when you look in your dog's eyes?
What do you think your dog is thinking when he looks in your eyes?
What is your favorite thing about your dog right now?
Is there anything you would change about your dog right now?
Is there anything you would want to stay the same?
What are your dog's silliest quirks and habits?
What are your dog's greatest talents?
What are your dog's favorite toys?
What are all the nicknames you have for your dog?
How did your dog become your best friend?

How did you become your dog's best friend?

Write a job description for your dog:

> *What "position" does she hold and what is the job title?*
> *What are her essential duties and responsibilities?*
> *What are the education requirements for this position?*

Pretend your dog is hiring you for a job and write the job description:

> *What "position" would you hold?*
> *What are your essential duties and responsibilities?*
> *What are the education requirements for this position?*

What goals do you have for your life together?

Now that we have looked at why you have your dog, let's figure out what, exactly, you got when you got that dog.

3

THE INNER GAME OF DOG

Question: What is the fastest way to determine the sex of a chromosome? Answer: Pull down its genes.

So, you got a dog—congratulations! Along with your dog, you got a *huge* packet of genes that have already determined much of your dog's physical appearance, physical skills, physical health, behavioral attributes, talents, and personality. Your dog is, essentially, a GMO: a genetically modified organism. She is the culmination of thirty thousand years of genetic modification—courtesy of your own ancestors—who originally performed that genetic modification by selective breeding to produce certain behavioral traits that they, the humans, found useful. As a result, your dog carries with her many inborn physical and behavioral traits that, frankly, may fit better with a lifestyle that many dog owners in the developed world don't have anymore—therefore, she may be instinctually eager to perform jobs that you no longer have any use for, and probably has a physique tailored to some obsolete physical task. In the previous chapter, you examined why you chose your dog—in doing so, did you choose her because of her breed? Or, if you have a mixed-breed dog, because of the breed you thought she appeared to be? Have you noticed that your dog does certain things that you never taught her to do, and that it can be hard to stop her from doing those things? Are these instincts the ones you expected when you chose your dog's breed? Or are there a few you didn't expect—maybe even a few that are complicating your life? The point here is that understanding what your dog's powerful innate aptitudes are can help you entertain your dog—

and yourself—in a constructive, not destructive, manner. Your dog's aptitudes, or talents, are either very obvious, or simmering somewhere just under the surface—and they need to be discovered and used, just like your ancestors used your dog's ancestors' instincts. All dogs living today carry with them lots of traits passed down to them, but they can really be boiled down to just two: the desire to please humans and the ability to perform a job. Luckily, you, just like your ancestors, can use the first trait to make the second one happen. And, believe it or not, this will help your dog live better and live healthier—and could even help your relationship. Let's examine your dog's physical and behavioral inheritance—but, first, Genetics 101.

39 AND YOU

We have all heard of chromosomes, and most of us know that humans have twenty-three pairs. You may not know, however, that dogs actually have thirty-nine pairs, and, you may or may not know what chromosomes really are. Chromosomes are thread-like structures located inside the nuclei of animal and plant cells. There are two types: coiled and linear. Ours and our dogs' are linear. Chromosomes are made of protein and a single molecule of *deoxyribonucleic acid* (DNA), and each one is crucial to the process that ensures DNA is accurately copied during cell division. Chromosomes are interesting because of their coiled shape, which keeps DNA tightly wrapped around other spool-like proteins (*histones*). Without the coils, DNA molecules would be too long to fit inside the cells—amazingly, if all of the DNA molecules in a single human cell were unwound from their histones and placed end to end, they would stretch six feet!

For an organism to grow and function properly, cells must constantly divide to produce new cells to replace old, worn-out cells. During cell division, it is essential that DNA remains intact and evenly distributed among cells. In humans and most other complex organisms, one copy of each chromosome is inherited from the female parent and the other from the male parent. There is a constricted region near the center of chromosomes known as the *centromere*, and this area helps to keep chromosomes properly aligned during cell division. *Telomeres* are repetitive stretches of DNA located at the ends of linear chromosomes which protect the ends of chromosomes in a manner similar to the way the tips of shoelaces keep them from unraveling. In many types of cells, telomeres lose a bit of their DNA every time a cell divides. Eventually, when all of the telomere DNA is gone, the cell cannot replicate and it dies—and this, by the way, is why anti-aging research is focused on keeping those little shoelace tips intact. Some anti-cancer research is focused on the same area for a different reason—the chromosomes of malignant cells usually do not lose their telomeres, helping to spur the uncontrolled growth that makes cancer *cancer*.

Each molecule of DNA has four amino acids. Dogs have 2.4 billion of these amino acids, which, when combined in sequences, make up thousands of genes. Although dogs have a higher number of chromosomes than do humans, dogs have fewer genes overall. Researchers sequencing the canine genome have identified around nineteen thousand dog genes compared to the twenty-five thousand or more genes in the human genome. This research has also shown that all domesticated dogs are genetically very similar—there is only a 0.2 percent difference in the genomes of all the dogs worldwide. Dogs do make the most of that lower number of genes—dogs are believed to have more physical and behavioral variations than any mammal on Earth. This is even more amazing when you consider that all of the diversity in the appearance and behavior of dogs has developed only within the last two hundred years!

But if they have fewer genes, how is it possible that a single species, *canis lupus familiaris*, could evolve so quickly? Body size in dogs, for example, can range from three to three hundred pounds, and is thought to be caused by a small variation in *a single gene* (the *insulin-like growth factor* [IGF-1] gene).[1] The area on the DNA where this gene (and genes governing other physical features such as muzzle length, coat characteristics, relative leg length, body proportion, and ear floppiness) has been found to be very prone to mutations, and dogs have many more of these mutations than other species.[2] It is hypothesized that this is why many genetically based physical characteristics and behavioral traits have evolved so quickly in dogs. Then, once humans began selectively breeding certain dogs in order to obtain dogs with a certain appearance or temperament, the process really sped up! However, selective breeding in a species that reproduces so rapidly (twice a year) has come to illustrate the law of unintended consequences: *an*

*intervention in a complex system tends to create unanticipated and of-
ten undesirable outcomes.* Humans have stimulated an explosion of diversity in a species that isn't really all that diverse, and then we have
taken the members of individual groups within that species and bred
them very closely over a very short time to produce certain traits. This
has led to some wonderful effects—great beauty, for one, and amazing
talents such as herding or retrieving—but also some not-so-wonderful
traits such as inherited health problems.

Genetic factors are involved not only in congenital malformations
(conditions with which an animal is born), but also metabolic disorders,
disorders of immune function, disorders associated with aging, and cancer. Many tests are now available to test dogs for a single-gene inheritance of 145 diseases, and the number of tests available will undoubtedly increase greatly over the next few years. Although purebred dogs are
at higher risk for these types of health problems, mixed-breed dogs can
get them, too, depending on the genetic background of their predecessors. That being said, the genetic background of a dog only tells what
could happen in terms of health and behavior, not necessarily what *will*
happen, since both of these factors are also affected by that dog's environment and experiences. That's where you and I come in. But where
did dogs, and the individual breeds, come from in the first place?

DANCING WITH WOLVES

Domesticated dogs, as a species, have been around for anywhere from
eighteen thousand to thirty-two thousand years. Genomic research has
also shown that dogs did indeed evolve from wolves, and this molecular
data suggests that dogs separated from wolves 10,000 to 135,000 years
ago—these are obviously very wide ranges. This issue has been undergoing heated debate since the time of Darwin—the different estimates
vary by the methods used to determine the dog/wolf split, and the time
and location of domestication by humans. Interestingly, only a small
number of genes is responsible for the difference between dogs and
wolves—it appears that only 0.04 percent of the canine genetic structure has changed from that of wolves.

Many researchers believe that domesticated dogs arose in the Middle East or Asia from wolves that began to follow human agricultural

settlements because the wolves learned that these settlements, and their waste, were a source of food. Other researchers believe that European hunter-gatherers domesticated dogs from wolves in Europe before agriculture was even developed. Recent DNA evidence taken from the bone of a five-thousand-year-old dog unearthed in Ireland suggests that both theories may be correct. Dogs may actually have been domesticated twice—once in Europe, and once in Asia, although it appears that the European line died out, and that all modern dogs are descended from the Asian line. [3]

Now we know more about *how* domesticated dogs developed (although there is still much research to be done), but what about *why*? Brian Hare, the author of *The Genius of Dogs*, has proposed that dogs domesticated themselves, without intentional human intervention at first, through natural selection: since wolves normally would have avoided human settlements, a subset of ancient wolves that were less afraid of humans, as well as less aggressive toward them, would have survived and reproduced not only because they had more food, but also because the less aggressive ones were not killed off by humans. [4] He calls this "survival of the friendliest," in which each generation of these dog progenitors became friendlier and friendlier. At some point, humans recognized how useful these creatures were for protection, hunting, and herding, and perhaps, dogs even had a role in human evolution—the groups of humans that lived with these dog progenitors, who benefited from the dogs' protection and the better food supply they helped the humans acquire, may have been better able to survive and reproduce. Eventually, dog domestication became intentional, with certain dogs, who had certain behavior traits and body types, being selected for by humans that needed certain jobs to be done.

Dogs that were good at understanding what the humans wanted, and thus were better at that job, would have been selected for breeding while those that were not would have been culled. The domesticated dog family tree started developing limbs that specialized in protection, herding, hunting, and, eventually, companionship, and these breed "clusters" of dogs of different shapes, sizes, and skills began at least three thousand years ago. The limbs on that family tree have sprouted many, many branches over the years because of increasing human needs for greater specialists within the groups of dogs—some herding dogs, for example, were developed to nip at the heels of cows and drive them in a certain direction. Other herding dogs were selected because they, working in groups, could contain a flock of sheep within a certain area, becoming a sort of "living fence" for the shepherd. Hunting dogs diverged into several groups: some hunting dogs were preferred because they were fast, could run down prey, and then would corner it, without killing it themselves, until the slower humans came to kill it. Other hunting dogs were valued and bred for their ability to track prey by its scent trail. Still others were chosen for their ability to indicate to humans where prey, such as a bird, were hiding, then flush the prey out of hiding so it could be killed, and finally bring the prey back to a human. Sounds like humans got lazier and lazier as we, and dogs, evolved, doesn't it?

Genetically, there are two major groups of dogs: one group that shares more genes with wolves, and one group that shares fewer genes with wolves. Members of the first group, the so-called ancient group, are found throughout the world, and this suggests that the evolution of dogs from wolves occurred in various places at various times. These dogs are: the *Afghan Hound* and the *Saluki* (from the Middle East); the *Basenji* (from Africa); the *Akita*, the *Chow Chow*, the *Dingo*, the *New Guinea Singing Dog*, and the *Shar-Pei* (from Asia); and the *Siberian Husky* and the *Malamute* (from the Arctic, and which are the only ones that show genetic evidence of interbreeding with wolves).[5] Members of the second group, the so-called European group, which share fewer genes with wolves, are basically all the other breeds we now recognize. Although members of the first group can be genetically distinguished from the members of the second group, it is harder to genetically distinguish members of the second group from each other, as most of their evolution has only taken place over the last few hundred years. However, some researchers, through further genetic analysis, have been able to divide the European dogs into four groups, although, as more and more canine genomic research occurs, the groupings shift occasionally:[6]

1. *Mastiffs and Terriers*—Examples include: Boston Terrier, Staffordshire Bull Terrier, Glen of Imaal Terrier, Jack Russell, Briard, Australian Terrier, Yorkshire Terrier, Cairn Terrier, West Highland White Terrier, Scottish Terrier, Mastiff, Bullmastiff French Bulldog, Miniature Bull Terriers, Boxer, Bulldog, Newfoundland, Golden Retriever, Flat-Coated Retriever.

2. *Herding dogs and sighthounds*—Examples include: Belgian Sheepdog, Belgian Tervuran, Collie, Border Collie, Shetland Sheepdog, Kuvasz, Ibizan Hound, Italian Greyhound, Whippet, Greyhound, Irish Wolfhound, Scottish Deerhound, Borzoi, Old English Sheepdog, Pembroke Welsh Corgi, Cardigan Welsh Corgi, Australian Shepherd.

3. *Mountain types*—Examples include: St. Bernard, Rottweiler, Great Dane, Bernese Mountain Dog.

4. *Modern*—Examples include: Pomeranian, Chihuahua, Pekinese, Shih Tzu, Brussels Griffon, Pug, Papillion, Miniature Pinscher, American Cocker, English Cocker, English Springer Spaniel, Cavalier King Charles Spaniel, Irish Water Spaniel, Brittany, German Short-haired Pointer, Bassett Hound, Beagle, Bloodhound, Petit Basset Griffon Vendeen, Dachsund, Havanese, Standard Poodle, Toy Poodle, Doberman Pinscher, Great Schnauzer, Standard Schnauzer, German Shepherd, Portuguese Water Dog.

I would never have expected some of these dogs to be in the same groups—this probably represents the influence of humans at that time still primarily breeding dogs for certain functions, rather than appearance, but beginning to want dogs with multiple talents. For example, the ancestors of Border Collies would have had herding instincts from the herding side of the family tree, but also great stamina for running from the sighthound part of the family tree. Because humans later took the members of the groups and bred them for appearance, the modern versions of these groups look very different from each other, but still might have some overlap in terms of their instincts for certain things.

You can see, therefore, that humans and dogs have historically— really prehistorically—had a mutually beneficial relationship. We chose dogs that wanted to please us, and exploited that trait—not in a bad way—to get them to perform certain jobs for us. In return, we fed them and cared for them, and they basically fed us and cared for us, too. But, somewhere along the way, about two hundred years ago, the *form* of dogs began to be valued, for reproductive selection, over their *function*. The appearance of individual types of dogs—the color of their coat, the length of their fur, the shape of their face, the position of their ears, the beauty of their movement—began to be used as a criterion for selec-

tion, instead of the talent. Most notably, certain jobs that were historically given to dogs required a certain physical type and, therefore, selection for appearance was not completely capricious. The dogs that are
now known as Neapolitan Mastiffs, who were used by Alexander the
Great in battle, needed to be large and intimidating, whereas the ancestors of the modern Welsh Corgi, whose job was to nip at the heels of
cattle, needed short legs to weave in and out between the cattle's legs
without being kicked. English Bulldogs, with their protruding lower
jaw, flat nose, and powerful neck muscles, were selected for the sport of
bull-baiting since they could clamp onto the muzzles of bulls and hang
on for long periods, while still breathing through their noses which
stuck out less than their jaws.

Groups of closely related domestic dogs, with a similar appearance
and characteristic traits, were thus developed from specific foundation
breeding stock into what we now call the individual dog breeds. Whether the domestic dog species benefited (or not) after humans began to
select them more for their appearance than for their abilities is a matter
of opinion—a case in point being the aforementioned Bulldog breed.
Fortunately, these dogs stopped being used for bull-baiting when the
sport was banned in England in 1835, and, once their function as a
breed was no longer being exploited, began to be valued for their appearance in the show ring. The physical traits that made them Bulldogs
originally—short nose, flat face, big head with powerful neck muscles,
and a small body—became progressively more exaggerated as time
went on, and the modern English Bulldog has a myriad of potential
health problems mostly related to the difficulty in getting enough oxygen through their very narrow nostrils and convoluted air passageways
in the nose, throat, and lungs. Their large heads and narrow pelvises
make natural birth nearly impossible, and most Bulldog puppies must
be delivered via C-section. Unfortunately, they also have the highest
incidence of hip dysplasia of any other breed, making arthritis even at a
young age almost inevitable. On a positive note, however, the breed's
fierce, bull-baiting temperament has been traded out for a docile, good-
natured, friendly personality, making English Bulldogs wonderful companion dogs that have enriched the lives of many dog owners. In addition, great efforts are being made by Bulldog breeders to reduce the
health problems, so, hopefully, the English Bulldogs of the future will
enjoy better health during a longer life.

Despite the fact that many types of dogs had already been developed by humans over the millennia, the actual concept of dog breeds dates only to the accurate documenting of pedigrees by the English Kennel Club, which was established in 1873 in an effort to mimic other stud book registries for cattle and horses. This placement of some dogs in specific breed categories, and excluding others, required standards regarding appearance, personality traits, and historical lineage. The trend among dog owners to value beauty over talent spilled over to the United States, and the Westminster Kennel Club Dog Show, which continues to this day, began in 1877 after the National American Kennel Club was established the year before. The National Greyhound Association was the first organization in America to encourage breeders to produce dogs with a specific goal in mind, but, initially, the goal was not appearance but racing speed. In 1882, this organization began to require that all racing dogs be registered in their studbooks before they were eligible to race, thus setting a new, at that time, trend for American and Canadian dog breeders: registration and proof of canine ancestry.

In 1884, a group of thirteen breed clubs (ten American clubs and three Canadian clubs) founded the American Kennel Club (AKC). The thirteen founding AKC breed clubs pledged "to do everything to advance the study, breeding, exhibiting, running and maintenance of purity of thoroughbred dogs." The AKC continued to grow and recognize other breeds—as of 2012, the AKC has recognized 177 separate breeds of dogs and has categorized them into eight groups, seven of which are based on the original purpose of the dog: *sporting, hound, working, terrier, toy, non-sporting,* and *herding.* Those dog breeds that did not fit into these seven groups were put into an eighth group: *miscellaneous.* Currently, there are many other breed registries, which recognize many of the same breeds registered by the AKC, but some that are not—overall, there are about four hundred recognized dog breeds worldwide.

What do all of these breed registries do? A breed registry places a breed into the appropriate category, called a group, and, then, some groups may be further subdivided. A dog is said to be purebred if the dog's parents were purebred and if the dog meets the standards of the breed, as established by the breed registries and the breed clubs for that breed. New breeds can be accepted into breed registries if it is represented by a sufficient number of individuals that have similar

physical and behavioral features, if they come from a select set of ancestors who had the same characteristics, and if they can be demonstrated
to reliably transfer those specific characteristics over generations. An
individual dog is identified as a member of a breed through proof of
ancestry, using genetic analysis or written records of ancestry, called
studbooks. The recognition of distinct dog breeds is not maintained by
any scientific organization, and the standards of the different independent breed registries can be inconsistent, and, therefore, so can the
purebred dogs they promote—maybe even the one you bought. Some
breed registries are very strict in their requirements that registered
breeders demonstrate, through genetic testing or medical certifications
(available for hips, elbows, hearts, eyes), that they are breeding healthy
dogs. Other breed registries have health standards but have no requirements for their documentation—accordingly, breeding for health is left
up to the ethics, and the consciences, of the breeders. And then there
are the breed standards for appearance, personality, and behavioral
traits, which are all subjective and certainly in the eye of the beholder,
or breeder, or judge.

PRETTY IS AS PRETTY DOES

Certain physical features of a breed go in and out of style and can
change greatly through close breeding in just a few generations. This
can happen with behavioral traits as well. After all, selection of dogs for
certain jobs has always required that those dogs displayed behaviors
that made them good at those jobs. Dogs used for herding and hunting
needed to have a strong enough prey drive to want to follow prey, but
not so strong a prey drive that they ate the prey before their humans
arrived to kill it. Herding dogs, who worked at a distance from their
humans, needed to use more eye contact and vocalizations to communicate with them than retrieving dogs, who needed more physical contact
(that explains a lot about my Golden Retrievers). Dogs selected for the
guarding of flocks needed prey drives that were even more suppressed,
and also needed to work independently without any contact with their
humans at all.

A skill at certain behaviors which were selected for by humans may
have led to the inheritance of certain personality characteristics, such as

independence or clinginess, within a given breed or, more specifically, within certain bloodlines. There is strong evidence that certain dog personality traits are inherited, as are some human personality characteristics. In humans, approximately 30 to 50 percent of the personality differences observed among humans are thought to be affected by genes. In dogs, studies have shown that activity, impulsivity, aggression, and fearful behavior are at least partly inherited.[7] Molecular geneticists have located certain gene variants in dogs that are associated with some behavioral traits, although it is important to emphasize here that these variants are *associated* with these traits—association does not mean that they are *caused* by them.

PRETTY IS AS PRETTY . . . DOESN'T?

This research helps show that, in spite of eons of selective breeding, a given purebred dog may or may not display the characteristic behaviors associated with her breed, and, within a breed, some members are more skilled in certain things than other members of the same breed. Some of this variation in behavior could be due to different dogs within a breed having different genetic sequences due to inherited mutations, but some of the variation could also be due to which genes in some dogs are turned on and which genes in others are turned off. This is the area of study in genetics called "epigenetics" and this variation in gene activity can be affected by environment, lifestyle, and age, and once those factors have changed the gene activity, those changes can then be passed to future generations. An example of this is maternal stress: fetuses carried by mothers that are stressed, which leads to an increase in the mother's blood level of the stress hormone cortisol will have changes in their own cortisol receptors, which can then be passed on to their own offspring, and then their offspring's offspring, even if none of them had stress during pregnancy. Changes in gene activation can also occur postnatally, and emotional and nutritional stress during an individual's life are common causes. In humans and rodents, this phenomenon has been associated with hyper-reactivity, meaning that the affected individuals respond to stress more extremely. In dogs, this may change the way certain dogs behave under stressful conditions, and may affect the ability of some dogs to learn if the environment in which they are being trained is too distressing to them.

This could have been the reason that the Golden Retriever I adopted in vet school, Ezra, had trouble learning to play and retrieve—his laboratory dog mother or grandmother was probably stressed during pregnancy, causing some genes to be activated or inactivated, which caused changes in Ezra's stress hormone receptors. He was, for his whole life, hyper-reactive to noises as well as any changes in his world, which made learning—and life—difficult for him. Ezra illustrates that *intent*, in terms of original purpose for a dog breed, and *reality* don't always line up in an individual member of that dog breed. Ezra, as a purebred Golden Retriever, *should* have displayed these characteristics as listed by the AKC for this breed: outgoing, confident, playful, friendly to people, anxious to fetch balls all day long. He was certainly some of those things—sweet, nonaggressive, loving—but he never displayed one iota of retrieving instinct and was much more comfortable with as few people or other dogs as possible. His breed-related instincts, as created by his forebears' original purpose did not match his personality, and his personality won out. This is why it is helpful, if you want to truly understand what your dog is capable of throughout her life, to see how her instincts, as bestowed upon her by her breed or breeds, fit with her personality. If you can recognize both her gifts and her limitations, if any, your lives together will be much easier—and healthier.

PURPOSE VERSUS PERSONALITY

In human psychology, *personality* is defined as "an individual's distinctive pattern of behavior, feeling and thinking that is consistent across time and situations." Animal behaviorists define personality, very generally, as consistent behavior over time in different contexts. For humans, many personality tests have been devised for many different reasons. They are used to diagnose psychological problems, to evaluate the effect of therapy, to look for changes in personality, to screen job applicants, and, like the one I have taken for my job, to see who will work best with whom. Most are self-assessments based on research using large numbers of people, and, to an extent, are scientifically validated, although they are limited by the accuracy and the honesty of the people answering the questions.

For animals such as dogs, personality testing is done, in part, to predict a dog's behavior in different situations in the future. Measuring behavior is about all we've got in animal personality testing, since we obviously can't question our subjects about what they are thinking and feeling as we can during human personality tests. However, several personality tests for dogs have been devised—these are based on owner or researcher observations and are difficult to scientifically verify since behavior in dogs is affected by experience and governed by thousands of genes, and controlling these variables to know the accuracy of these tests is impossible. Part of the problem is also that "science" requires measurement—and "measuring" personality traits such as intensity, aggression, and fearfulness is difficult. That being said, some aspects of the personality tests that have been devised by animal behaviorists might be useful in your evaluation of your dog's personality.

Human personality is often described by using the "The Big Five"— which are five broad domains of personality that appear to be consistent over a wide range of ages and cultures. These five factors are: *openness, conscientiousness, extraversion, agreeableness*, and *neuroticism*. These, obviously, would not be directly applicable to dogs, but the model has been so useful in the evaluation of human personality that similar domains of canine personality have been sought.

Researchers in Sweden found four personality factors to be stable in a standardized behavioral test that involved 13,097 dogs.[8] They were: *playfulness, curiosity/fearlessness, sociability*, and *aggressiveness*. Stable, in this case, refers to the traits being displayed repeatedly by a given dog over time in different circumstances. Interestingly, the breeds of the dogs were not predictive of the traits they displayed. One of the researchers' objectives was to find out whether there was a difference in personality between members of a given breed if they came from a line of dogs that were bred to perform the historical function of the breed (working dog use), or from a line of dogs bred simply for their appearance (show dog use). This was, in part, meant to see how we modern-day humans are currently making the dog species evolve. They found that selection for working dog use tended to produce dogs that were more playful or more aggressive. Selection for show dog use tended to produce dogs that were less aggressive, but less playful and curious in potentially threatening situations. They were also more fearful in both social and nonsocial situations. Another interesting finding was that dogs from the most popular breeds were more playful and more social, suggesting that the lines that are winning at the shows may not be "in line" with the kinds of dogs people want, and that a new selection pressure is at play: besides selection for function and form, there is now, by dog owners, selection for companionship. If, by the way, the selection pressures could also include good health, the dog species would benefit, and veterinarians would not be as busy.

Although this personality test showed some interesting and surprising results about the personality of dogs, the personality test itself is unwieldy and definitely is not something to try at home with your own dog—one part of the test had the handler firing a gun to measure the reactivity of the dog! Other parts of the test involved throwing a human-like dummy in front of the dog and having people dress like ghosts to see how the dog would react. Although this may be a good test to measure your dog's behavior on Halloween, it may not be possible or useful at other times.

Another research group, in Hungary this time, devised a questionnaire for the assessment of dog personality that is useful for our purposes in this book. It was also adapted from the Big Five and included the traits of: *trainability*, *boldness*, *calmness*, and *sociability*. There were seventeen questions within the four categories, and owners were asked to answer using a three-point scale, with 1 meaning "did not agree" and 3 meaning "agreed strongly." The test was published in the German *Dogs* magazine as well as on the magazine's website, and a total of 14,004 questionnaires were collected from dog owners, but the researchers were only interested in purebred dogs, so, in the end, 5,733 questionnaires from ninety-eight breeds were analyzed with the most frequent breed being Labradors.

The traits were analyzed in terms of the conventional dog groups: herding, hounds, working, sporting, nonsporting, terrier, and toy. The researchers also analyzed the effect of the breeds' genetic relatedness in some behavior traits, so they categorized them into the five clusters mentioned earlier: the wolf-like (ancient) cluster, the Mastiff-Terrier cluster, the herding/sighthound cluster, the mountain cluster, and the modern (hunting) cluster. When analyzing the conventional dog groups, no breed-related differences were noted regarding calmness and dog sociability, but there were significant differences in trainability and boldness. Herding dogs were reported to be more trainable than hounds, working dogs, toy dogs, and nonsporting dogs, while sporting dogs were reported to be more trainable that nonsporting dogs. Terriers scored higher on boldness than both hounds and herding dogs. When the genetic clusters were analyzed, no differences in calmness and dog sociability were found, but the ancient cluster was less trainable than the herding/sighthound and hunting cluster. The Mastiff-Terrier cluster was bolder than the ancient breeds, the herding/sighthound cluster, and the hunting breeds.

I just threw a ton of information at you—and I wouldn't be surprised if you were thinking: *Hey, this stuff is interesting* (I hope you are thinking that), *but* why *do I need to know it?* Well, if you use all this information, put together by hundreds of researchers in the fields of canine history, genetics, and behavior to figure out the personality of your own dog, you can then use all that to provide a custom-tailored healthy, active lifestyle for your dog, that suits her personality and temperament, and fits you both. Why is this important for you and your dog? It's the old nature versus nurture dichotomy—your dog's genetic code, both physically and behaviorally, is already determined, but whether or not some genes are turned on or off are determined by her environment, her nutrition, and her stress—*that* is the nurture half of the equation—and that depends on *you*. Your dog's genetics and epigenetics have created a unique set of behavioral and physical traits, and, while some may line up with her breed or breeds, some may not. This means that you need to figure out her individual personality and physical capabilities, so that you can tailor her environment to allow her to express her own distinctive pattern of behavior in a healthy way, which may reduce stress and increase health for both of you. So, now that we have deconstructed the domestic dog species and dog breeds, let's deconstruct your own dog (figuratively) and then put all that information back together to help you understand "The Inner Game" of *your* dog, giving her the freedom to be what she really is.

4

THE INNER GAME OF *YOUR* DOG

Fortunately, most children learn to walk before they can be told how to by their parents. —Zach Kleiman, *The Inner Game of Tennis*

You've seen how dogs, as a species, have been defined by humans over the years in multiple ways—function, breed, appearance, behavior, and genetics. Since your dog is the pinnacle of dog evolution to this point, we could use that same sort of information to define, and hopefully understand, your own dog. He arrived at your doorstep with some ancestral and experiential baggage, based on his genes, his inborn personality traits, and his experiences. Without understanding who your dog is, and what he is, you won't really know how to direct him through life. After all, you two will be together longer than many people remain married, so you might as well get to know each other. Think about the things you put in his Time Capsule at the end of chapter 2—some of those questions were observational in nature, but some were aspirational. What is it you want out of life with your dog? What are your goals for him? These next sections will help you define how well your dog fits in with those plans and what you need, if anything, to do to keep him on a positive pathway through life.

LOOK AT YOUR DOG'S *FUNCTION*, OR JOB, IN YOUR LIFE

Companionship

- inside the house—for company during quiet times
- outside the house—for company during walks or gardening

Protection

- yourself
- your home

Therapy

- yourself
- someone else

Exercise Partner

- walking
- running

Sports

- Hunting

  - retrieving
  - pointing
  - flushing
  - nose (scent) work
  - herding

- Competition

  - conformation dog shows
  - working dog trials

- dog sports

Other—anything else you put down in the job description you created at the end of chapter 2.

LOOK AT YOUR DOG'S *BREED*

Since most people are familiar with the AKC, and their website, AKC.org, has lots of useful information about the 177 breeds recognized in the United States, that is a good place to start. Keep in mind that the breed descriptions contain the somewhat idealized version of that breed, and, so not to offend any particular breed enthusiasts, tend to tip-toe around certain potentially troublesome characteristics of a breed. Their interactive website contains much more information about each breed than could possibly be contained in this book, but a basic summary follows.

Look at these AKC groups, and see which group your dog is in, or, for mixed-breed dogs, which one you think your dog is in. Look at the history and "typical" behaviors, but remember not to be "breedist"—since your dog might not be consistent with the described breed characteristics, look at the other breed descriptions and their specialties, to see if he is the nonconformist type and has other, unexpected talents. Write down the breed of your dog (or what you think your dog is), the jobs that breed was intended to do, plus any personality characteristics from any of the breed groups that you think describe him. See how well these historical functions of your dog's breed, and the personality characteristics you have noted for him, line up with the jobs for which you hired your dog, as listed in the first section. Look also for any unknown talents your dog might have, based on his ancestry.

By the way, if you own a dog with a mixed genetic ancestry, consider completing a DNA test. These are both useful and fun. There are several companies that offer these, and there are two types: one that uses DNA collected by you at home and sent back by mail, using a cotton swab rubbed inside your dog's cheek, and one that uses blood collected by your veterinarian. The blood-test type is more expensive but also more helpful in some ways, since it compares your dog's genes to a bigger database of dog DNA and also gives you information about health problems that might be related to your dog's genetic background. You may want to check with your veterinarian to see if this test is offered at your veterinary clinic or which test is recommended.

Sporting Group

The (recent) historical purpose of this group of dogs was to locate, flush, and retrieve game for hunters, and there are four subgroups:

- *Pointers* do what their name indicates, and often stand rigid and silent, indicating the location of prey.
- *Spaniels* flush game, meaning they will rush at prey to make them come out of hiding.
- *Setters* find and point at game, and also flush game.
- *Retrievers*, well, retrieve.

General behavioral traits (and some of the words I found online to describe this group):

- bred to work closely with people and are eager to please and easy to train
- high stamina, do well with running and hiking activities, as well as sports such as agility
- excellent swimmers

Breeds in this group include: American Water Spaniel, Brittany, Chesapeake Bay Retriever, Clumber Spaniel, Cocker Spaniel (American and English), Curly-Coated Retriever, English Setter, English Springer Spaniel, Field Spaniel, Flat-Coated Retriever, German Shorthaired Pointer, German Wirehaired Pointer, Golden Retriever, Gordon Setter, Irish Setter, Irish Water Spaniel, Labrador Retriever, Pointer, Spinone Italiano, Sussex Spaniel, Vizsla, Weimaraner, Welsh Springer Spaniel, Wirehaired Pointing Griffon.

Hound Group

The historical purpose of this group was to track down and chase game for hunters. Within this group, there are two subspecialists, each with their own behavioral characteristics:

Scent Hounds:

- use their extremely acute sense of smell to track prey
- once on the scent, tend to focus on that one task and exclude all others
- are very active when "on the job," very chill when they are "off the clock"
- have a somewhat deafening "bay" of a bark that can carry for very long distances

Breeds in this group include: American Foxhound, Basset Hound, Beagle, Black and Tan Coonhound, Bloodhound, Dachshund, English Foxhound, Otterhound, Petit Basset Griffon Vendeen.

Sighthounds:

- use their amazing speed to run prey down
- will be off like a rocket, and travel nearly as far, if they see something move at a distance
- may not be great at resisting the impulse to chase cats, cars, and bikes or anything that moves fast

Breeds in this group include: Afghan Hound, Basenji, Borzoi, Greyhound, Harrier, Ibizan Hound, Italian Greyhound, Irish Wolfhound, Norwegian Elkhound, Pharoah Hound, Rhodesian Ridgeback, Saluki, Scottish Deerhound, Whippet

Working Group

This group of dogs includes those that were originally bred for guarding people, property, and livestock, and pulling carts or sleds. As such, many of these dogs are very large and very strong. Some of the oldest breeds, such as Mastiffs, were actually bred by the Romans to hunt lions.

General behavioral traits:

- protective of their family and property
- can be suspicious of people not within their family unit
- can have low-indoor activity, in contrast to their high-outdoor activity needs

Breeds in this group include: Akita, Alaskan Malamute, Anatolian Shepherd Dog, Bernese Mountain Dog, Boxer, Bullmastiff, Doberman Pinscher, Giant Schnauzer, Great Dane, Great Pyrenees, Greater Swiss Mountain Dog, Komondor, Kuvaz, Mastiff, Newfoundland, Portuguese Water Dog, Rottweiler, Saint Bernard, Samoyed, Siberian Husky, Standard Schnauzer.

Terrier Group

These dogs were bred to hunt and kill vermin, which is defined as any animal considered to be a nuisance to people, their crops, and property. They tend to be small in stature but large in attitude, and, as the AKC website says: "They are always eager for a spirited argument."

General behavioral traits (for some reason, there are a long list of words to describe this group—maybe because of that "big" personality!):

- feisty
- bold
- independent-minded
- tenacious
- plucky
- fearless
- confident
- alert
- spirited
- entertaining
- active

Breeds in this group include: Airedale Terrier, American Staffordshire Terrier, Australian Terrier, Bedlington Terrier, Border Terrier, Bull Terrier, Cairn Terrier, Dandie Dinmont Terrier, Irish Terrier, Jack Russell Terrier, Kerry Blue Terrier, Lakeland Terrier, Manchester Terrier, Miniature Bull Terrier, Miniature Schnauzer, Norfolk Terrier, Norwich Terrier, Scottish Terrier, Sealyham Terrier, Skye Terrier, Smooth Fox Terrier, Soft Coated Wheaten Terrier, Staffordshire Bull Terrier, Welsh Terrier, West Highland White Terrier, Wire Fox Terrier.

Herding Group

These dogs were bred to control the movement of other animals, usually livestock such as sheep and cows. They do this in a variety of ways, depending on the breed—some do this by either nudging or nipping at their legs to encourage movement in a certain direction, while others will stand in front of the livestock and stare them into submission. The herding instincts in these dogs will often generalize to the herding of people and, especially, their children, along with some nipping at their heels, which is generally not well received.

Here are words used to describe members of the herding groups, along with their general behavioral traits:

- workaholic
- driven
- intense
- energetic
- smart
- confident
- industrious
- resourceful

Breeds in this group include: Australian Cattle Dog, Australian Shepherd, Bearded Collie, Belgian Malinois, Belgian Sheepdog, Belgian Tervuren, Border Collie, Bouviers des Flandre, Briard, Canaan Dog, Cardigan Welsh Corgi, Collie, German Shepherd Dog, Old English Sheepdog, Pembroke Welsh Corgi, Puli, Shetland Sheepdog.

Toy Group

All the dogs in this group are smaller versions of a diverse array of larger dogs and were meant to be small enough to be held in a person's lap or arms. Their behavioral characteristics are as varied as their ancestors and generalizations, except about size, are hard to make. Since they were selectively bred to be good companions, most of them do that job very well, although that trait can be overlaid with some traits inherited from their original breed. Some are very protective of the people that hold them, and can be snappy, while others are accepting of all strangers and are indiscriminate cuddlers.

Breeds in this group include: Affenpinscher, Brussels Griffon, Cavalier King Charles Spaniel, Chihuahua, Chinese Crested, English Toy Spaniel, Havanese, Italian Greyhound, Japanese Chin, Maltese, Miniature Pinscher, Papillon, Pekingese, Pomeranian, Toy Poodle, Pug, Shih Tzu, Silky Terrier, Toy Manchester Terrier, Yorkshire Terrier.

Nonsporting Group

This group of dogs was formed because they do not share common behavioral traits with other breeds; therefore, they are also very diverse and difficult to describe in general terms. Some were bred for sports or purposes that no longer exist, such as (fortunately) bull-baiting (Bulldogs) or the untangling of fishing nets (Poodles). Others have evolved so far from their ancestors that they can't be grouped with the modern representatives of that original breed anymore—for example, Dalmatians evolved from herding dogs to run alongside coaches, but were also bred for their elegant looks. The breeding pressure for appearance won out and modern Dalmatians do not generally display herding behavior.

Breeds in this group include: American Eskimo Dog, Bichons Frise, Boston Terrier, Bulldog, Chinese Shar-Pei, Chow Chow, Dalmatian, Finnish Spitz, French Bulldog, Keeshond, Lhasa Apso, Lowchen, Poodle, Schipperke, Shiba Inu, Tibetan Spaniel, Tibetan Terrier.

LOOK AT YOUR DOG'S *PERSONALITY*

Get a little more specific by taking an adaptation of the Hungarian researchers' temperament test for your dog. Using a scale of 1 to 5, with 1 indicating strong disagreement, and 5 indicating strong agreement, see if you think the following statements describe your dog. Write the numbers down on a separate sheet of paper, along with the four traits (trainability, boldness, calmness, dog sociability), and then, at the end, add up all the scores within each group. The high numbers indicate your dog's strongest personality traits.

Trainability

Is your dog . . .

- ingenious/inventive, when seeking a hidden food or toy?
- intelligent/learns quickly?
- very easy to warm up to a new toy?
- good at understanding what is expected during playing?
- interested in lots of things besides eating and sleeping?

Boldness

Is your dog . . .

- never cool or reserved?
- never unassertive or aloof when unfamiliar persons enter your home?

Calmness

Is your dog . . .

- calm, even in ambiguous situations?
- rarely stressed?
- emotionally balanced, not easy to rile?
- cool-headed, even in stressful situations?
- seldom anxious and uncertain?

Dog Sociability

Is your dog . . .

- rarely the instigator of fights with dog family members?
- ready to share toys with dog family members?
- seldom bullying toward dog family members?
- able to get along well with dog family members?

LOOK FOR POTENTIAL *PROBLEMS*

Now let's see if your dog has any problems that you might need to seek help for, and which might interfere with certain activities, using the same 1–5 scale (adapted from the Dog Personality Questionnaire [DPQ] developed at the University of Texas):[1]

Stranger-Directed aggression

Does your dog act aggressively . . .

- when approached directly by an unfamiliar male adult while being walked or exercised on a leash?
- when approached directly by an unfamiliar female adult while being walked or exercised on a leash?
- when approached directly by an unfamiliar child while being walked or exercised on a leash?
- toward unfamiliar persons approaching your dog while it is in your car?
- when an unfamiliar person approaches you or a member of your family at home?
- when an unfamiliar person approaches you or a member of your family away from home?
- when mail carriers or other delivery workers approach your home?
- when strangers walk past your home while your dog is in your yard?
- when joggers, cyclists, roller skaters, or skateboarders pass your home while your dog is in your yard?

• toward unfamiliar persons visiting your home?

Owner-Directed Aggression

Does your dog act aggressively . . .

• when verbally corrected or punished by a member of your household?
• when toys, bones, or other objects are taken away by a member of your household?
• when bathed or groomed by a member of your household?
• when approached directly by a member of your household while eating?
• when food is taken away by a member of your household?
• when stared at directly by a member of your household?
• when stepped over by a member of your household?
• when a member of your household retrieves food or objects stolen by your dog?

Stranger-Directed Fear

Does your dog act anxious or fearful . . .

• when approached directly by an unfamiliar male adult while away from your home?
• when approached directly by an unfamiliar female adult while away from your home?
• when approached directly by an unfamiliar child while away from your home?
• when unfamiliar persons visit your home?

Nonsocial Fear

Does your dog act anxious or fearful . . .

• in response to sudden or loud noises?
• in heavy traffic?

- in response to strange or unfamiliar objects on or near your sidewalk?
- during thunderstorms?
- when first exposed to unfamiliar situations?
- in response to wind or wind-blown objects?

Dog-Directed Fear or Aggression

Does your dog act aggressively . . .

- when approached directly by an unfamiliar male dog while being walked or exercised on a leash?
- when approached directly by an unfamiliar female dog while being walked or exercised on a leash?
- toward unfamiliar dogs visiting your home?

Does your dog act anxious or fearful . . .

- when approached directly by an unfamiliar dog of the same or larger size?
- when approached directly by an unfamiliar dog of a smaller size?

Separation-Related Behavior

Does your dog display . . .

- shaking, shivering, or trembling when left or about to be left on his own?
- excessive salivation when left or about to be left on his own?
- restlessness, agitation, or pacing when left or about to be left on his own?
- whining when left or about to be left on his own?
- barking when left or about to be left on his own?
- howling when left or about to be left on his own?
- chewing or scratching at doors, floor, windows, and curtains when left or about to be left on his own?
- loss of appetite when left or about to be left on his own?

Attachment or Attention-Seeking Behavior

Does your dog . . .

- display a strong attachment for a particular member of your household?
- tend to follow a member of household from room to room about your house?
- tend to sit close to or in contact with a member of your household when that individual is sitting down?
- tend to nudge, nuzzle, or paw a member of your household for attention when that individual is sitting down?
- become agitated when a member of your household shows affection for another person?
- become agitated when a member of your household shows affection for another dog or animal?

Trainability

Does your dog . . .

- return immediately when called while off-leash?
- obey a sit command immediately?
- obey a stay command immediately?
- fetch or attempt to fetch sticks, balls, and other objects?
- seem to attend to or listen closely to everything you say or do?
- seem slow to respond to correction or punishment?
- seem slow to learn new tricks or tasks?
- seem easily distracted by interesting sights, sounds, or smells?

Chasing

Does your dog . . .

- act aggressively toward cats, squirrels, and other animals entering your yard?
- chase cats if given the chance?
- chase birds if given the chance?
- chase squirrels and other small animals if given the chance?

Excitability

Does your dog overreact or become excitable . . .

- when a member of your household returns home after a brief absence?
- when playing with a member of your household?
- when your doorbell rings, or just before being taken for a walk?
- just before being taken on a car trip?
- when visitors arrive at your home?

Pain Sensitivity

Does your dog act anxious or fearful . . .

- when examined or treated by a veterinarian?
- when having claws clipped by a household member?
- when groomed or bathed by a household member?

This information in the last two sections could help you when thinking about whether your dog might enjoy or train well for activities inside or outside your home, especially those that involve other people or other dogs. It can also give you an idea of things to work on in training—your dog's behavioral traits may be consistent over time, but are not completely unbendable. I, for example, have always been a bit (maybe more than a bit!) messy and somewhat disorganized, but, because I eventually got a job and got married, was faced with the need to change my behavior—I wish I could say those inclinations were not still things I battle against, but I can say that, with effort, they have gotten less severe over the years. If you find that your dog has certain predispositions that could preclude involvement in certain activities that you want to do, don't assume you can't do them—consult a veterinary behaviorist or a trainer to see if you can modify those tendencies. Bring the results of your dog's personality tests along—they will be a valuable resource for the consultant.

SPEAKING OF TRAINING . . .

A veterinary behaviorist is a veterinarian who has completed a residency program in the field of veterinary behavioral medicine. These specialists in veterinary behavioral medicine have both the medical and behavioral knowledge to evaluate your dog to determine if there is a medical component to the behavior, and they can formulate an appropriate treatment program that includes behavioral modification and, if needed, medications. These specialists are not trainers, but have a different type of expertise. A dog trainer also uses behavior modification to change a dog's behavior by teaching a response to cues or commands.

There are many types of training, but the keys to successful training lie in understanding a dog's personality, the use of consistent communication, and the accurate timing of positive reinforcement. Training methods, unfortunately, still exist that involve punishment, and many involve establishing dominance over a dog in an attempt to mimic the dominance hierarchy of dogs. Actual behavioral research has shown that, although a dominance hierarchy exists among groups of dogs, humans are not included within that hierarchy—because dogs, not surprisingly, recognize that humans are not dogs. If a human suddenly decides to roll a dog over on her back to imitate what some dogs do to establish dominance over another dog, the surprised dog can feel threatened, and then might decide that the best defense is a good offense—and bite. I have had several clients, who listened to a famous trainer, and were physically injured that way—and, unfortunately, the injury was not just physical—damage was done to the trust that the dogs placed in the owner, and vice versa. According to the evolutionary anthropologist mentioned earlier, Brian Hare, research on free-ranging dogs shows that the "pack leader" is the one that has the most friends—this probably goes back to the original wolves that evolved into the dog species because they were the friendliest. Much of the dominance-type training taught by some trainers was derived from research into wolf pack–dominance hierarchies. But dogs, despite being descended from them and sharing much DNA, are not wolves—they are a separate species because they had a different set of selection pressures.

Here is some advice on how to select a trainer (adapted from the American College of Veterinary Behaviorists' website, dacvb.org):

- Call, interview, and, ideally, observe a trainer prior to hiring. Take the time to see for yourself how the trainer treats the dogs in the classes or consultations.
- If the trainer you are considering uses any of the following methods, you should run the other way and pick another trainer:

    - The equipment recommended for basic obedience includes or is focused on choke collars, prong collars, or shock collars. Trainers who ban head collars of any kind may rely unduly on force.
    - The trainer instructs you to manage your dog's behaviors by pinching toes, kneeing the dog in the chest or abdomen, hitting the dog, forcibly holding the dog down against their will, constantly yelling at the dog, frequently yanking the collar, or using prong, choke, pinch or shock collars or electronic stimulation.
    - The trainer believes most or all training is about encouraging the person to be "alpha" and teaching the dog to "submit."
    - The trainer explains that most dog behavior, for example, jumping on people, occurs because the dog is trying to be "dominant."
    - A trainer recommends "alpha rolls," "scruffing," "helicoptering," "choking," or any other painful or physical methods as a means of "training" or modifying behavior.
    - Please note that having initials after a trainer's name (i.e., has graduated from a training program) is *not* a guarantee of a trainer who will not engage in these practices.

These last four sections should have given you four different ways to look at your dog's multifaceted personality. The behavioral traits that you discovered in each section may have lined up well with each other—or they may not have matched well at all—but they all say something about your dog, and what kind of game she got.

ONE LAST THING—LOOK AT *YOURSELF*

You may not want to, but you should. After all, you and your dog are two halves of a relationship—since you now know the other half pretty well, you owe it to your dog to understand yourself a little, especially in regard to your own behavior toward your dog in certain situations. In studies of the influence of human personality's effect on the choice of human partners, there is consistent evidence that the more similar two individuals are, the higher the attraction between them. Apparently, this "similarity-attraction hypothesis" holds true for humans who choose certain dog partners.

A study done on Hungarian and Austrian dog owners and their dogs showed significant correlations between owners and their dogs on all five personality dimensions of neuroticism, extraversion, conscientiousness, agreeability, and openness.[2] Also, many experts in behavioral disorders in dogs agree that owner's attitudes toward their dogs contribute to a variety of behavior problems. More specifically, the owner's personality can be associated with certain behavior problems: in one study, owners of aggressive dogs were reported to be less stable, more disciplined and more tense than owners of nonaggressive dogs: this, however, could have been because the owners were overly protective of their dogs and didn't socialize them well.[3] In another study, anxious, neurotic owners may make their dogs more nervous because they don't behave consistently with them.[4] Before you get too worried about your own personality shortcomings in regard to your dog, please keep in mind that I have included this information to illustrate that you do have the ability, unintentionally or intentionally, to influence your dog's own personality and behavior—but you need to learn about yourself first.

This is the "Big Five" personality test. I have listed the questions that are on it, and you may just want to read through them for self-reflection, but, if you want to know how you actually score in the personality traits of openness, conscientiousness, extraversion, agreeableness, and neuroticism, take the test online at a variety of websites. Just use the search term: "big five personality test" and you will find several—if you feel comfortable filling them out and submitting the answers to a third party. Here is the link to one of those websites: outofservice.org/bigfive (I have also provided this link on howtoageproofyourdog.com).

Directions: The following statements concern your perception about yourself in a variety of situations. Indicate the strength of your agreement with each statement, using a scale of 1 to 5, with 1 indicating strong disagreement, and 5 indicating strong agreement. On a separate piece of paper, write down the question number and the number that denotes the strength of agreement/disagreement.

I see myself as someone who . . .

1. is talkative.
2. tends to find fault with others.
3. does a thorough job.
4. is depressed, blue.
5. is original, comes up with new ideas.
6. is reserved.
7. is helpful and unselfish with others.
8. can be somewhat careless.
9. is relaxed, handles stress well.
10. is curious about many different things.
11. is full of energy.
12. starts quarrels with others.
13. is a reliable worker.
14. can be tense.
15. is ingenious, a deep thinker.
16. generates a lot of enthusiasm.
17. has a forgiving nature.
18. tends to be disorganized.
19. worries a lot.
20. has an active imagination.
21. tends to be quiet.
22. is generally trusting.
23. tends to be lazy.
24. is emotionally stable, not easily upset.
25. is inventive.
26. has an assertive personality.
27. can be cold and aloof.
28. perseveres until the task is finished.
29. can be moody.

30. values artistic, aesthetic experiences.
31. is sometimes shy, inhibited.
32. is considerate and kind to almost everyone.
33. does things efficiently.
34. remains calm in tense situations.
35. prefers work that is routine.
36. is outgoing, sociable.
37. is sometimes rude to others.
38. makes plans and follows through with them.
39. gets nervous easily.
40. likes to reflect, play with ideas.
41. has few artistic interests.
42. likes to cooperate with others.
43. is easily distracted.
44. is sophisticated in art, music, or literature.
45. is politically liberal.
46. has high self-esteem.

Now that you know your own personality a little better, see how what you do could be affecting your dog. Think about the subconscious cues you are giving him, and the ways you could be reinforcing some of the behaviors you don't want. And if you do ever consult a trainer or veterinary behaviorist, your own insight into your own personality strengths could be very helpful in creating a training plan for your dog.

In this chapter, you learned a lot about your dog and yourself, and how you fit together. You may adore your dog, and, of course, he adores you—but it's also possible that, by this time, you have figured out a few things that are (or are not) working in your relationship. After all, love at first sight does not always lead to happily ever after—acquiring a new life partner, and learning how to live together harmoniously, can be wonderful, but, admit it, occasionally awful, at the same time, whether that life partner is human or canine. In many ways, people choose canine life partners in the same way they choose the human ones. In human dating, some people just fall in love at first sight after a chance encounter, others go on dating websites and fill out a detailed questionnaire about the type of person they are, the type of person they want, and the type of relationship they seek. In canine "dating," some people fall in love at first sight at a pet store or shelter, others do extensive research into the breed they want. However, the big difference is that humans can always turn down a second date with an incompatible human, or break up after a while, and both parties will usually survive to go on to other relationships. It's not that way when someone adopts a dog—breaking up is definitely hard to do, since breaking up with a dog involves finding that dog a new home or giving him up to a shelter.

In my experience, most dog owners who find themselves paired with a dog that is incompatible with their own personality or lifestyle will do one of two things—they will just keep the dog even if it makes both the owner and the dog unhappy, *or* they will do something to help their square peg of a dog fit into the round hole of their life. Hopefully, this information will keep the first thing from happening because it has made the second thing possible. After all, relationships are like any work of art—they are made of individual components that fit together, and enhance each other, to make something whole that is better and more beautiful than the components are when they are apart. Relationships, as well as works of art, also require dedication and effort every bit as much as they require inspiration and talent, and will benefit from a step back, an objective inspection, and a tweak here and there, to make them become masterpieces.

5

GETTING TO KNOW YOU

Outside of a dog, a book is man's best friend. Inside a dog, it's too dark to read. —Groucho Marx

LET'S GET PHYSICAL

My goal in this book is to train you, the owner, to learn and perform the tasks needed to ensure, as much as is possible, a long, healthy, and comfortable life for your dog. One useful habit to establish throughout the life of your dog is the performance of a regular—say, once monthly—head-to-toe-to-tail physical exam. That way, you will learn what is normal for your dog so you will be aware of changes soon after they occur, and then you can alert your veterinarian. I do very thorough physical exams on my patients every time I see them, but I may miss a new skin bump on a thickly furred Sheltie. A dog owner who performs a routine body check once monthly, or during daily grooming, will certainly notice that new bump and can point it out to me. You don't need to go to vet school to learn how to do this type of exam—you just need to be attentive and diligent about doing it throughout the life of your dog—this will certainly serve you and your dog well, particularly in the senior years.

The kind of exam I recommend starts with the head (mouth, teeth, ears, eyes, and neck), moves down the body (back, chest, and abdomen), takes a quick peek under the tail, checks the tail itself, moves down the legs, checks the feet and toes, as well as the pads and the areas between the pads, while checking the condition of the skin and fur throughout. This sounds as if it would take a lot of time, but shouldn't, once you and your dog get accustomed to its routine occurrence. It is very important to start this type of thing as young as possible, so that your dog will become used to it, and not object when you check such areas as the teeth, ears, and feet. In addition, your puppy or young adult's teeth, skin, body, and weight should be pretty healthy, so, if you learn what is normal at that stage of life, you can recognize when it is not. Don't forget to reward your dog with small, delectable treats frequently throughout the process, both in puppyhood and throughout adulthood, although the attention and semi-massage your dog will get from you during the exams will themselves provide much of the positive reinforcement—for both of you. Here's what to do:

Head

Mouth

- Pull up your dog's lips starting in the front where the tiny teeth (incisors) and "fang" (canine) teeth are, and check for brown tartar buildup and red, swollen, or receded gums, as well as discolored (gray or purple) or broken teeth. Continue this type of exam along the sides of the mouth, and don't forget to check the teeth way in the back by pulling the corners of your dog's lips open, then back toward the back of the head and slightly up toward the ears.
- Check the gums as well as the lips themselves for bumps and sores. You will also inevitably be aware (sorry!) of any bad breath, which can be a sign of periodontal disease. One of the benefits of starting this exam in puppyhood is that you will become aware of how many teeth your dog has, and, will know, without even completing a veterinary dentistry class or ever looking at an anatomy book, what normal dog teeth look like—as they should be perfect in your puppy once the adult teeth come in, after about six months of age. If you are brushing your dog's teeth (hopefully often!), you will also be aware of changes in the mouth as they occur over the years.

Nose

- Look at the nostrils for crusty nasal discharge, and along the sides of the nostrils as well on top of the nose for sores or scaly, thickened skin.

Eyes

- Check the eyes for yellow or green discharge—a little clear mucus in the corners of the eyes is OK but very thick and plentiful mucus discharge, especially if it has a yellow or green color, is abnormal.
- Pull up the upper lids of the eyes to look at the "whites" (*sclera*) of the eyes—they should indeed be white, with a few tiny, pink blood vessels visible—but widespread redness in that area is abnormal. If your dog's eyes are a little saggy in the lower lids (common in breeds such as Labs and Bassett Hounds, for example), there may be a little redness noted inside the lids themselves. This concerns some of my clients until they are shown that pink is the normal color of the inside of the eyelids, and that the sagginess of the lower lids of some dogs just makes that normal pink color more visible. I then teach them to look at the sclera (above the colored part of the eye and under the upper lids) which is where the signs of eye irritation or infection more reliably show up.
- While you are looking at the lower lids, look toward the inner (toward the nose) corners of the eye for the "third" eyelids (the *nictitans*)—these may be normally colored pink, white, or black. They may be more or less visible depending on how alert or awake your dog is, but, when dogs are sick or dehydrated, the third eyelids are more visible and cover more of the eyeballs in the inner corners.
- Check the clear surface of your dog's eyes (the *cornea*) with a flashlight, looking for white or brown deposits, and note, just very generally, if both pupils are equal in size and shape.
- Look for cloudiness inside the eyes, beyond the pupils.
- Check the upper and lower lids and their edges for bumps.
- Note if your dog seems to be squinting in one eye more than the other.
- If you have a long-haired dog or a terrier, check to see how much the hair growing around the eyes may be obscuring the vision—sometimes this hair can be very long, and it functions like blinders on a

horse. This is particularly hard on older dogs who may already have some visual changes and coordination issues.

Ears

- Check the ear flaps (*pinnae*) for swelling, bumps, scabs, and loss of fur.
- Look down inside the ears (in the ear canals, using a flashlight) for brown debris, redness, or odor. Look for hair growing around and inside the ear canals, as well as mats and foreign objects tangled in the fur.

Neck

- Run your hands along the side of the neck and under the jaw to check for lumps and swellings. You may actually feel some lumps in the upper part of the neck and under the jaw that may be normal salivary glands, but let your veterinarian know where they are, so your vet can tell you whether they are normal or not.

Body

Chest

- Run your hand along the ribcage on both sides to see if you can feel the ribs easily without too much "padding" and to look for a little greater breadth in the chest/ribcage area (when looking down from above the back) compared to further toward the back legs. Being able to feel the ribs, without being able to actually see them, and then seeing whether there is a tapered decrease in body width as your hands move along the sides toward the back legs demonstrates whether or not your dog's weight is ideal, or not so ideal, for your dog's frame size. Dogs come in so many breeds, and so many sizes even within breeds (and then there are the mixed breeds!), that it is difficult to recommend the one right weight for every dog, and it is more useful to see how the weight looks on the individual dog. (This is called "body condition scoring" and most veterinarians include this as part of their routine exams.) Also become aware of your dog's basic body contour as you run your hands along the sides, top and underneath part of the chest and abdomen, so you will recognize any new lumps or bumps under the skin layer or on top of it.

- Rest the palm of your hand along the left side of your dog's ribcage, just behind and slightly below the elbow of the left front leg to measure what your dog's heart rate and rhythm are while resting. The normal heart rate for dogs is between 70–160 beats per minute, and tends to be on the lower end of this range for the larger dogs (60–140 beats per minute for giant breed dogs), and on the higher end for the smaller dogs (up to 180 beats per minute for toy breed dogs). There is some normal variation in the rate and rhythm that occurs with breathing (called *sinus arrhythmia*) and this means that the heart speeds up slightly as the dogs take in a breath and then slows down slightly as the breath is let out. Again, the value of checking this is to know what's normal, and what *not* to worry about, so you will then recognize what is abnormal and what to consult your veterinarian about.

Abdomen/Back

- Run your hands along the sides, and underneath the area of the body beyond the end of the ribcage and toward the dog's back end so you can feel the tapering of the waist (hopefully, at least *some* tapering is there!) as well as a slight "tuck" in the underneath part of the abdomen, which also should be visible when the body is viewed from the side—this is to be expected if the body weight is ideal, and striven for if the body weight is too high. A "gut" hanging down toward the ground is as bad for dogs as it is for humans, so know if it is there or not!
- Feel the skin and the layers below that for lumps and bumps, then move your hands up to the back, then all the way down to the base of the tail, and along the tail itself. It is very easy to miss new bumps on the tail, as that is not a common place that people pet their dogs. Notice if your dog winces at all, or if the skin twitches or "crawls" as you feel along the back bones—these are sometimes signs of pain.
- While you are "down there" (the way most of my clients refer to the anal and genital areas in their dogs), lift up the tail and check for any swelling, bumps, or redness in the skin around the anus and under

the base of the tail. For female dogs, check the skin around the vulva (the area below the anus where the urine comes out) for redness and discharge, and note any odor you detect at a distance. Also check the areas under and around all of the nipples for firm lumps below the surface (female dogs get breast cancer, too). For male dogs, check the tip of the penis for redness and excessive discharge—a small amount of yellowish mucus seen on the tip of the sheath or prepuce (the equivalent of the foreskin) is normal.

Legs

Joints and Muscles

- Run your hands down all four legs to see if there is any swelling in any particular area compared to the equivalent areas on the other legs. Get an idea of the thickness of the muscles over the shoulders and thighs as this can change with age, arthritis, and some neurologic conditions.
- Bend and straighten some of the joints (elbows, wrists, hips, knees) with the palm of your hand against the part of the joint that you are bending *away* from to get an idea of the flexibility of that joint as well as any "crunching" or crackling (called *crepitus*) in those joints. Decreased flexibility or crepitus can be an indicator of arthritis and "popping" in the knee joint can be an indication of a kneecap (*patella*) that doesn't want to stay in place (*luxates*).
- Watch your dog get up from lying down, and note any hesitation or extra effort that seems needed.
- Observe your dog walking, trotting, or running and note any limping or bobbing of the head (a subtle sign of soreness in one of the front legs).

Feet, Toes, Claws, and Pads

- Examine the toes for swelling, and check the claws for cracking and excessive length. Long claws are not only hard on your floors, but are also hard on your dog, too—very long claws actually make it difficult for a dog to walk normally, and long claws are also candidates for breakage down into the quick—broken (avulsed) nails are painful, bleed profusely, and can get infected. While you are there, trim the tips of the nails if they are long.

- Look at the pads on the underside of the feet for cracking or peeling (common in the summer when a dog walks on very hot pavement) as well as cuts, punctures, and bumps. Warts and corns occur on the feet of dogs just like they do in humans, and they can be just as uncomfortable to walk on.
- Feel the skin between the pads and between the toes (on the top as well as the underside of the feet) for burrs stuck in the fur and bumps on the skin.
- If you have a long-haired dog, check the length of the fur growing from the areas between the pads—if it is long, the fur can cover the pads while the dog is walking and take away the traction provided by the rough surface of the pads—dogs will slip and slide on tile or hardwood floors and get injured, just like a human running on those surfaces in socks! This is especially hard on older dogs that have lost some muscular strength and flexibility. Have your groomer or veterinarian's staff clip the fur short between the pads.

Skin and Fur

- Throughout your head-to-toe-to-tail exam, pay attention to the skin—look for redness, scabs, dandruff, and lumps or bumps.
- Look for reddish-brown discoloration of the fur—this can indicate that your dog has been licking the skin. The discoloration is due to a pigment from the saliva, called porphyrin, which builds up on the fur over time with repeated licking.
- If you find bumps, you should have your veterinarian check them, but my clients often can't find the bumps once they get into the office (the skin of dogs is pretty loose and mobile and a bump can appear to be in one location when the dog is in one position, and seem to be in a different location when the dog is in another position). It helps to mark the fur near the bump with a little nail polish or a dab of color from a magic marker—just don't use dark red nail polish like one of my clients did—when the dog walked in the clinic, the staff rushed over to him in horror, thinking he had been stabbed in multiple places! You can also keep track of the various lumps and bumps that will develop over the years by marking them on a

sketched outline of your dog's body. I have provided one with the physical exam checklist shown here, and it can also be printed from the website howtoageproofyourdog.com.

THE INSIDE STORY

Now that you have systematically checked over the outside of your best friend, time to check the inside—even though Groucho thinks it is too dark to read in there, you can "see" a lot, if you think about it in the right way. Look over your physical exam inventory and quickly "review the systems"—this is a tool that human health-care providers use when they examine their patients. This list of questions, arranged by organ system, is designed to uncover symptoms that a patient might not know are important indicators of disease. Human health-care providers have the luxury of completing this pretty easily, since most of their patients can talk and answer their questions! Pediatricians and veterinary health-care providers don't have it quite so easy and have to rely on the observations of their patients' caretakers for the review of systems—and that is where you, the "parent" of your pet, come in. As you look at the physical findings you have compiled during your exam, think about how well those particular areas are functioning. Go from head to toe to tail again, just very generally, and consider the following areas.

Head

- Brain: Seriously, how is your dog's brain doing? Any changes in his ability to do tricks, play games, solve problems, remember where you have hidden shoes that you don't want him to have? Any increase in anxiety or aggression? Any restlessness at night? How alert is he? How responsive to you? Is he more or less affectionate with you or other members of the family?
- Mouth and Neck: Think about your dog's appetite. Is your dog still eating as fast and as much as he once was? Finishing all the food? Leaving lots of crumbs, as if he is not chewing as well? Swallowing OK? Dribbling water more than he used to? Do you think that your dog has any trouble bending his neck down to eat or drink from his bowls? Does he have trouble getting to his bowls?

- Eyes: Think about your dog's vision. Can your dog still see annoying squirrels at a distance? Can he still snatch a treat out of the air with accuracy? Is he misjudging distances or falling more than in the past?
- Ears: How is the hearing? Is your dog still greeting you when you get home, or does he remain asleep until you get closer or touch him? Still hearing the quietest, teeniest little crackle of a treat package while upstairs under a blanket?

Body

- Chest or Heart: How is the breathing? Louder than before, heavier, more effort? Any coughing or gagging? Is your dog able to exercise for as long as before? Does he want to turn around and go home during walks earlier than he used to, or lie down suddenly during activity?
- Abdomen and "Down There": Urinating or defecating more or less often than before? Larger or smaller amounts? Any straining or extra effort? Any accidents? Although it is not exactly appetizing to watch your dog urinate or defecate, watch closely every so often—dogs have to assume a very specific position to defecate (hunched back, legs under the body) and dogs with weak or arthritic back legs can't always maintain that position long enough to empty the rectum. If this happens every day, stool can build up and these dogs will sometimes have accidents even though they are still perfectly housetrained.

Legs

- Joints and Muscles: Is your dog slow at the end of a long walk? Any limping? Any dragging of the feet? After a lot of exercise, is he agile while moving, but stiff after rest, and then become flexible again after moving around a bit? If you have a smartphone, filming your dog in slow motion while walking, trotting, or running can really show you—and your vet— subtle changes in gait that could be important and easy to miss when your dog is moving at his normal speed. Also, many dogs that limp at home will not limp at the veterinary clinic—the excitement of the car ride and veterinary visit will cause your dog's adrenaline level to rise. This can mask pain, and therefore, limping. Having a slow-motion video of your dog's symptoms to show your vet can really aid your vet in making a diagnosis—and will look really impressive!

OK, so how was that for a crash course in vet school? I know that seems like a lot to remember, but if you use the list every month, it really won't take you long to go through it from memory and perform it quickly. It will help to look at the checklist and at figures 5.1 and 5.2, shown below. You can download copies of all three from howtoage-proofyourdog.com—save your results over the years in order to compile a lifelong home health record for your dog.

In figure 5.1, there is a basic outline sketch of a dog shown from both sides, so that you can draw in information about location of lumps and bumps, or to remind you of the location of areas of concern, so that you can show it to your veterinarian. In figure 5.2, you will find a Body Condition Scoring chart that will show you how to assess your dog's weight without needing a scale so that you keep track of your dog's Body Condition Score over the years when weight will inevitably, but possibly subtly, fluctuate.

Don't forget, this is an investment of time and attention that will help your dog age successfully and help *you* be your dog's first line of defense against health problems that may affect the length of your time together. John F. Kennedy once said something that I think applies to the effort and time that is needed to age-proof your dog: "There are risks and costs to action. But they are far less than the long range risks of comfortable inaction." All of this will take time, and perhaps some expense, but will pay off by giving you more time—together.

PHYSICAL EXAM AND REVIEW OF SYSTEMS CHECKLIST.

Mouth/Lips:

_____

_____

Teeth:

_____

_____

Nose:

_____

_____

Eyes:

_____

_____

Ears:

_____

_____

Neck:

_____

_____

Can feel ribs easily?
    Yes ___ No ___

Chest area wider than waist?

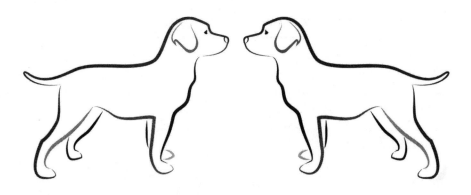

Figure 5.1.   Your Dog's Body. Thinkstockphotos.com/yod57.

Yes ____ No ____

Heart Rate:
        _____ beats per minute

Breathing Rate:
        _____ breaths per minute

Gut or Tuck:

_____

_____

Back:

_____

_____

Tail:

_____

_____

Skin/Fur:

_____

_____

Lumps and bumps:

_____

_____

Genital area:

_____

_____

Anal Area:

_____

_____

Right front leg:

_____

Left front leg:

_____

Right front foot:

_____

Left front foot:

_____

Right hind leg:

___

Left hind leg:

___

Right hind foot:

___

Left hind foot:

___

Changes in behavior/memory/playfulness?

___

Changes in vision or hearing?

___

Changes in appetite/water consumption?

___

Changes in breathing/panting?

___

Changes in urination/defecation?

___

Changes in energy level/stamina?

___

Changes in mobility/stiffness/limping?

___

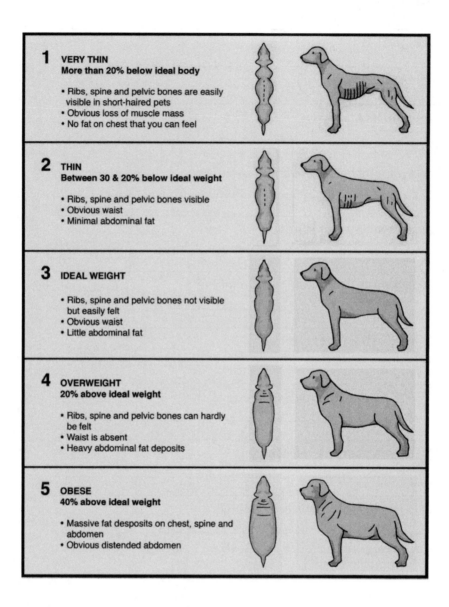

1 **VERY THIN**
More than 20% below ideal body

- Ribs, spine and pelvic bones are easily visible in short-haired pets
- Obvious loss of muscle mass
- No fat on chest that you can feel

2 **THIN**
Between 30 & 20% below ideal weight

- Ribs, spine and pelvic bones visible
- Obvious waist
- Minimal abdominal fat

3 **IDEAL WEIGHT**

- Ribs, spine and pelvic bones not visible but easily felt
- Obvious waist
- Little abdominal fat

4 **OVERWEIGHT**
20% above ideal weight

- Ribs, spine and pelvic bones can hardly be felt
- Waist is absent
- Heavy abdominal fat deposits

5 **OBESE**
40% above ideal weight

- Massive fat desposits on chest, spine and abdomen
- Obvious distended abdomen

Figure 5.2.   Dog Body Condition Scorecard. Illustration by Katy Murphy Ingle.

6

GETTING TO KNOW *ALL* ABOUT YOU

Equipped with his five senses, man explores the universe around him
and calls the adventure Science. —Edwin Powell Hubble

So what, exactly, is a "sense"? According to the Merriam-Webster Dictionary, a sense is "a specialized function or mechanism (such as sight, hearing, smell, taste, or touch) by which an animal receives and responds to external or internal stimuli." Dictionary.com defines a sense differently: "it is the feeling or perception produced through the organs of sight, hearing, smell, taste or touch." The key point of the second definition is the use of the word "perception"—which is itself defined as: "the organization, identification and interpretation of sensory information as provided by specialized sensors in the body in order to construct a mental representation of the physical world." In other words, one's *senses* provide raw data, while one's *perception* translates that data into meaning.

Imagine, for example, a tennis ball on the ground. The light reflected off the ball enters the eye and stimulates the retina, a layer coating the back of the eyeball that contains cells that are sensitive to light. This triggers nerve impulses that pass via the optic nerve to the brain, where a visual image is formed. The visual image that is formed depends on the visual apparatus possessed by each species of animal encountering that ball—the visual image that I form when I see that ball is quite different from the one my dog forms, as you will discover in this section. What that tennis ball on the ground actually *means* depends on the perceiver, since perception is influenced by learning, memory, and expectation. When I see a tennis ball on the ground, its meaning is something like "Here is something that I need to pick up before someone trips over it, like I did yesterday," while, when my ball-crazy Golden Retriever, Shrek, sees that tennis ball, its meaning to him is most likely something quite different. I will never really know what my dog thinks when he sees the ball, but I can guess his thoughts by his actions of running to the ball, picking it up, and bringing it back to me with a wagging tail! I doubt he is reacting to the memory of seeing me trip over the ball yesterday, thus picking up the ball to prevent me from doing so today. Rather, he remembers that I usually throw the ball when he picks it up and brings it to me.

The same ball triggered stimulation of both of our retinas, but the neural pathways within our bodies took the light hitting that ball, translated it not only into different mental representations of the ball, but also different interpretations of that sensory information. Interestingly, when I see an apple that has fallen off the kitchen counter to the floor, I know it is an apple and not a tennis ball—because of the way I sense color and the way I have learned, through memory and experience, to perceive "red, round object on the kitchen floor is most likely a fallen apple, not a tennis ball." Shrek, of course, sees another tennis ball—partly because he can't tell the difference in the colors of these round objects—but also because he perceives almost everything in terms of tennis balls. . . .

Why is this important? In these next few chapters, I will compare your senses of sight (vision), hearing (audition), smell (olfaction), taste (gustation), and touch (tactioception) to those of your dog. With this information, I want you to change *your* perception of your dog's perception of the world. *News flash*—it's not the same as yours! In a way, I want you to do the opposite of anthropomorphism, which is to give human attributes to animals. Anthropomorphism is from the Greek roots *anthropose* (human) and *morphos* (form). In fact, I invented a new word for this exercise—"caninomorphism" (from the Latin word for dog, *caninus,* plus *morphos*), which, for the purposes of this book, will mean to give your dog's sensory attributes to yourself, and to imagine what his perception of the world is. Besides being just plain interesting and maybe kind of fun, imagining the world from your dog's point of view—perceiving the world the way your dog does—can be useful in understanding some of your dog's behaviors, particularly as his senses of vision, hearing, smell, taste, and touch change with increasing age.

THE VISION THING

The sense of sight is a complicated and somewhat wondrous process that begins with light reflected off an object; this light passes through several specialized structures and is converted into impulses carried by millions of tiny nerves in the back of the eye, which are then gathered by the optic nerve to be sent to the brain for formation of an image. A change in any of the structures along this pathway can change the image received by the brain and can, therefore, interfere with perception.

As shown in figure 6.1, two structures are located in the outer, or front, parts of the eye which have the primary function of bending the reflected light rays to shrink the object's image and bring it into focus on the coating in the back of the eye; these are the *cornea*, which is a clear coating on the outermost layer of the eye, and the *lens*, located just behind the colored part of the eye, the *iris*. When the cornea is healthy, it is smooth, moist, and clear with a slight bulge in its center. It

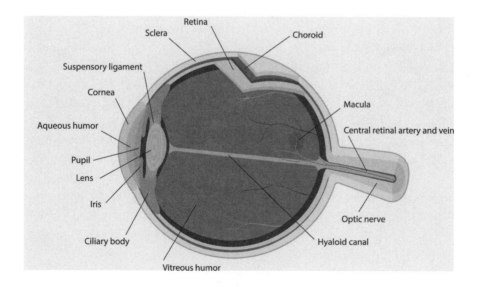

Figure 6.1.   The Eye. Thinkstockphotos.com/*oculo*.

does not just passively transmit light, like a window, but begins the process of bending it. When light rays hit a transparent body, like window glass, that is perpendicular to the surface of that body, they will pass through it without bending. If, however, the transparent body has a bulge or curvature to the surface, like the cornea, the light rays will change angles as they pass through it. This is how the cornea bends the light reflected off an object and starts the process of bringing it into focus on the retina. The cornea contributes 65–75 percent of the eye's total focusing power.

Once the light passes through the cornea, it then passes through an area called the anterior chamber, which contains a clear, gel-type substance called the *aqueous humor* that holds this space open and passively transmits the light. The iris's opening, the *pupil*, widens or narrows to adjust the amount of light that hits the lens just behind it. The *lens* is a clear, flexible, crystalline structure that actually changes shape, becoming thicker or thinner in response to the actions of the *ciliary body* (which is attached to the underside of the iris and produces the aqueous humor), to further bend the light and precisely focus the image on the back of the eye.

When an object is far from the eye, it is small relative to the eye, and the angle of the light reflected from it are nearly parallel to each other as they travel through the eye. However, when an object is close to the eye, it is relatively large, and the angles of the light reflected from it diverge from each other. For the image to be in focus on the retina, light rays from the near object must be bent more than those from the far object. The lens does this by assuming a more rounded shape when the viewer needs to look at an object near the eyes. The closer the object, the more the light will need to be bent, and the thicker and rounder the lens will have to become. The light then passes through another gel, the *vitreous humor*, which keeps the posterior chamber, and the eye, from losing its spherical shape, but does not bend the light.

After that, the light hits the retina, which is composed of millions of cells that are designed to receive the energy contained in the light. The retina converts this energy into electrical and chemical signals which are, in turn, gathered by the optic nerve and sent to the brain. One item to note—light rays emanating from the top and the bottom of the object move closer together as they approach the eye, and at a certain point, they actually cross and reverse, projecting an image onto the retina that is upside-down and reversed.

The retina is primarily composed of two types of photoreceptors: *rods* and *cones*. These cells each have a distinctive shape—hence their names—and distinctive functions. Rods are specialized to respond to dim light, and are found along the edges, or periphery, of the retina. They provide peripheral or side vision. Rods also allow the eye to detect motion. Cones are specialized to respond to light in different ways, and together are responsible for the perception of color. In humans, cones are found in the center of the retina, in an area called the *macula*, and the area within the *macula* where they most densely concentrated, the *fovea*, is a small depression in the back of the eye. The fovea is the target area for the light that started way outside the eye—it is the area upon which the light is most focused and where the visual image is clearest.

In dogs, a similar target area where the focused light is most focused is called the *area centralis*, although the photoreceptor cells have a pattern different than that of humans. For both species, the signals from the photoreceptor cells in the most superficial layer of the retina pass through two other deeper layers of nerves within the retina; these nerves detect contrast or changes within the image that indicate edges or shadows as well as other information about color. The signals are all sent to the *optic nerve*, which then routes them primarily to the *cerebral cortex* in the brain where visual perception is created.

This visual cortex, amazingly, contains a point-to-point map of the image that corresponds with the exact image that was focused on the retina—except that it turns the image right-side-up again! Plus, it receives two images—one from each retina—and it knits them together into one. Areas of the visual cortex are specialized to detect horizontal versus vertical orientation, the dimension of depth (by comparing slight discrepancies in position between the images received from each eye) and the edges of objects, all of which aid in the task of visual recognition. Some of the signals are sent to areas in the brainstem, which help with visual mechanics. One area, the *pretectum*, helps govern pupil size related to the intensity of the light; another area, the *colliculus*, helps the brain perceive a smooth image by stitching several still images together. Some information about image color, fine structure, contrast, and motion is processed in the *thalamus*.

To summarize, the eyes receive and transmit raw data, and the brain pulls out information about color, form, motion, spatial orientation; the information is then shaped by learning, memory, and expectation, and, in the end, visual perception occurs. And this happens with every bit of light bounced off every object during every fraction of every second that we, and our dogs, have our eyes open! What does that get us both? The ability to adapt to the continual shifts in our surroundings, and survive—whether it is by avoiding a collision while driving a car hurtling along at seventy miles per hour on a busy highway, or by successfully chasing and catching prey—or, at least, a bouncing tennis ball.

The differences in visual perception between humans and dogs start with differences in the raw data that the brain receives. In general, humans are stars in the areas of color perception and fine focus at close distances in bright light, while dogs excel at peripheral vision involving moving targets in dim light. This, of course, makes perfect sense given our respective evolutionary pathways and priorities for survival over the eons. However, awareness of this, and possibly trying to "see" like your dog will help you understand why he does not always see a treat on the floor a couple of inches in front of him, but can catch a treat with accuracy when it is tossed from the side to an equivalent distance near his face. It will also make you realize that dog toy and dog food manufacturers are really marketing to *your* color perception, not your dog's, when they come out with different colored toys and visually appealing dog food that looks like it has bits of green and orange vegetables in it. Like light, we are moving from the front of the eye to the back while we examine this.

Eye Position

The brain can judge the position and depth of objects based on the slight difference in position of the images sent to it from each eye. If an object is close to the eyes, the difference in the images will be great, but if an object is far away, the difference in the images will be small. Depth perception depends on this as well as on the width of each eye's visual field, which is the entire area that can be seen when the eye is directed forward, including that which is seen with peripheral vision. Where the two visual fields overlap, the depth perception is best. As shown in figure 6.2, the eyes of humans are on a plane even with the forehead, while those of dogs are more laterally placed toward the sides of the head. Dogs, therefore, have a wider field of view than humans, but there is less overlap between the visual fields of each eye. For humans, the visual fields of each eye overlap by about 140 degrees (this is called *binocular convergence*), but for dogs, there is only a thirty- to sixty-degree overlap. Better overlap means better depth perception, so humans win there, but wider field of view means better detection of objects in the periphery, such as predators or prey, so dogs win on that! The human binocular field of view is 180 degrees, while some dogs, such as Greyhounds and Whippets, have a field of vision up to 270 degrees, although broad-headed breeds with short noses, such as Pugs and Bulldogs, have a much narrower field of vision, as low as we poor humans at 180 degrees!

Interestingly, the depth perception of dogs varies by breed, since some breeds have a higher nasal bridge, which blocks some of the overlap of the visual fields, especially when the dog is not looking straight ahead. Some dogs have long or fluffy hair in the area around and in between the eyes, which can impair their binocular vision and depth perception. Whereas we can't change our dog's eye position or breed to improve depth perception, we *can* groom them so as not to impair it further. If you want to practice a little caninomorphism, you obviously can't move your eyes to the sides of your head to increase your visual field, but you can place a couple of fingers on the bridge of your nose to mimic a dog's high nasal bridge, or cup your hands around

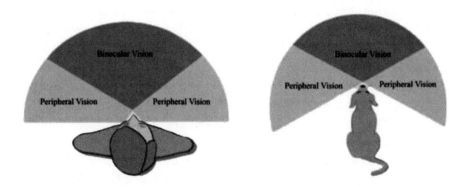

Figure 6.2. Comparison of the Fields of View of Humans versus Dogs. Illustration by author.

your eyes to simulate the impact of extra hair there—see how much of your visual field you lose, and how this impacts your depth perception?

The Cornea

The corneas of humans and dogs are actually fairly similar in their microscopic structure, but the overall corneal size is larger in dogs than in humans, allowing dogs to gather more light from their larger field of view and bend it further to focus on the retina. This feature also helps dogs see better in dim light. Interestingly, the thickness of the corneas of both species varies with the time of day—the cornea is normally thicker in the morning; it retains fluids during sleep that evaporate in the tear film while the eyes are open during the day. Humans with different ethnic backgrounds and dogs from different breeds have different corneal thicknesses. The average corneal thickness in humans is 0.55 mm, while in dogs the average is 0.64 mm.

The Iris and Pupil

The primary function of the iris is to control how much light gets into the eye, and it is embedded with muscles that widen or narrow the tissue gap in its center, the pupil. The pupils of humans and dogs have the same round shape, whereas in other species, like cats, they are more slit-shaped. The size of the pupil is governed by a sphincter muscle, which, when tightened, makes the pupil smaller, and by dilator muscles, which pull the iris in a circular fashion, pleating the iris tissue into folds. When the pupil is wide, more light enters the eye, and when the pupil is small, less light enters the eye, and the pupil continually makes adjustments in size to optimize vision based on the surrounding amount of light.

The size of the pupils in humans can vary from 1 mm to 9 mm, while dogs have a much smaller pupil size range of 3–4 mm, which means their pupils are always ready to receive as much light as possible. This is helpful for creatures that hunt at night, as they will see better in dim light, but this does lead to a bit of a sacrifice in visual acuity. When the pupil constricts, it limits the amount of light that hits the retina by blocking the light scattered by the edges of the cornea, and this makes the image projected on the retina sharper. If the pupil is limited in constriction, as it is in dogs, too much light will be allowed into the eye under bright circumstances; this leads to excessive light scatter, and the image will be blurred as a result.

The color of the iris in humans is much more varied than it is in dogs: most dogs have irises that are some shade of brown, probably for the purposes of camouflage. Eye color in dogs is genetically based, as it is in humans, and some breeds, such as Huskies and Australian Shepherds, have blue, or partially blue, irises. Iris color has aesthetic value—at least to humans—but has no effect on visual acuity.

The Lens

The degree to which the lens bends light, called *accommodation*, is dependent on the action of the ciliary body and its suspensory ligaments—these are tiny fiber "guy wires" from which the lens is suspended. It seems backward to me, but the lens becomes flatter and wider when the ciliary body relaxes and the suspensory ligaments contract to pull edges of the lens outward, and becomes rounder when the ciliary body contracts and the suspensory ligaments relax. Therefore, the ability of the lens to focus an image sharply on the retina depends on the clarity of the lens, the flexibility of the lens, the thickness it can achieve, the strength of the ciliary body and the tension of the suspensory ligaments. Humans, at least when they are young, have optimized all these factors for sharp vision at a wide variety of distances. However, as humans get older, the lens loses some of its flexibility, and it is unable to become as fat as it should to bend the light from a close object in order to focus it on the retina. This is called *presbyopia* and is the first rite of passage to middle age in humans, requiring people over the age of forty years old to buy reading glasses.

The dog lens, which is more spherical than the human lens, as well as stiffer, can't change its shape as easily. In addition, the dog lacks some of the groups of muscle fibers controlling lens shape that humans possess. The vision of most dogs, as related to the ability of their lenses to focus an image on the retina, is basically presbyopic—blurry at close distances. For the purposes of caninomorphism, if you are over forty and wear reading glasses, take them off to see what your dog sees at close distances. If you are younger than forty, there are several websites that show what presbyopia will look like for you in the future! Enter the search term "presbyopia simulation" and you will get several. Or go to howtoageproofyourdog.com to see what your dog sees. Reading—whether it be letters or facial expressions—matters a lot to humans in terms of survival; to dogs, not so much. It is the general shape and movement of prey, or of another predator, that determines whether life continues—or not.

The Eyeball

The diameter of the *globe*, or eyeball, of adult humans is relatively constant among the different sizes of humans and the different ethnic groups. The size of the globe varies less between different dog breeds than one might think, despite the vast difference in body size between a Saint Bernard and a Chihuahua. The size of a dog's eye can look misleadingly large or small to a human, as our judgment of eyeball size is affected by how much of the eye is covered by the lids—some breeds have more prominent-appearing eyes because their lids retract more than others.

Globe diameter has little effect on visual acuity—but globe shape, or length from front to back, has a huge effect on it. Ideally, the degree to which the cornea and lens bend the light reflected from an object will be exactly the amount needed to put the image in focus on the retina. However, if the eyeball is elongated from front to back, and, even if the cornea and lens do a great job of bending light from a distant object to focus the image, the image itself won't reach the retina, but will be focused slightly in front of it, and the image will be blurred. An object close to the eye will be slightly larger so its image will reach the retina and the image will be sharper. The ability to see near objects better than far ones is called near-sightedness, or *myopia*. The opposite happens when the eyeball is slightly short from front to back—an object close to the eye will be focused slightly behind the retina, so its image will be blurred, while an object far from the eye will be focused on the retina and will be clear. This is called far-sightedness, or *hyperopia*.

Among humans, there is great variation in eyeball shape and the tendency to be near- or far-sighted is genetically based. Those that have either condition must wear corrective lenses to bring images into precise focus on their retinas; the degree to which the focus must be changed by the lenses is measured in diopters, is a negative number for near-sightedness to be corrected, and a positive number for far-sighted-ness to be corrected. The most familiar measurement of human visual acuity is the Snellen fraction, which measures the ability of humans to distinguish between letters at a fixed distance of twenty feet. 20/20 vision is considered perfect for people; this means that a test subject can correctly identify letters from a distance of twenty feet compared to the average person with normal vision; a person with 20/30 vision iden-tifies letters correctly from a distance of twenty feet that the average person with good vision can identify from a distance of thirty feet, and so on.

This is, obviously, not a test that can be done on dogs. Tests that are done on dogs vary in methodology, including the use of behavioral responses, measurement of brain responses to visual stimuli, measure-ments of retinal stimuli to light, and responses to rotational movement, so estimates of visual acuity in dogs vary widely. These studies, taken together, indicate that most dogs have visual acuity of about 20/75, although near-sightedness appears to increase with age in dogs. There are some breeds of dogs that have a higher incidence of near-sighted-ness even as young dogs, and these breeds are German Shepherds, Miniature Schnauzers, and Rottweilers. Of the German Shepherds tested in one study, half were guide dogs and half were pet dogs—the pet dogs were much more near-sighted than the guide dogs, probably because those with near-sightedness had not done well in the training process and were kicked out.

Before you call your veterinarian to schedule an eye chart exam for your Rottweiler, however, it must be pointed out that there is no practi-cal way for you or your vet to precisely measure your dog's degree of near- or far-sightedness. A veterinary ophthalmologist can use an in-strument called a retinoscope to measure that—this is what is used in children who are too young to read an eye chart. This handheld instru-ment projects a beam of light into the eye—when the light is moved vertically and horizontally across the eye, the examiner observes the movement of the red reflex from the retina (the reflection of the light off the retina, which is mostly red because of all the blood vessels). The ophthalmologist then puts lenses in front of the eye until the movement stops and the power of the lens required to stop the movement indi-cates the lens strength needed to correct the vision. This is *not* some-thing your veterinarian will have—what will be used is an ophthalmoscope, which is used to look at the back of the eye, and has different lenses in it to change the focus for the user, not the patient. Veterinarians will sometimes do a crude test of vision on dogs suspected to have more severe visual deficits by moving something across the dog's visual field and seeing if the dog notices it.

The most common test veterinarians use is "the menace"—moving a hand toward the dog's eyes to see if he reacts by blinking, and the "cotton ball test," which involves tossing cotton balls across the dog's visual field. Cotton balls are used since, to humans, they don't have much color, don't have much odor, don't move much air, or make much noise when they hit the ground—but this test will give little information about mild visual changes. The other problem with this test is that dogs can smell, hear, or feel most objects that are tossed close to them, even cotton balls—it is hard to really know if they are seeing them with their eyes or sensing them in some other way. Another problem with this test is that it may test the dog's ability to sense motion more than it does visual acuity, and since dogs are very good at sensing motion, dogs that respond to this test may appear to have better vision than they do. Results have indicated that dogs that fail this test have a visual acuity of 20/400—if those dogs were people, they would be legally blind!

By the way, there are glasses available for dogs—really goggles—but they don't contain lenses to correct for poor vision; the lenses are really intended for eye protection and are an excellent idea for dogs under certain circumstances, and for the same reasons humans use them. If you and your dog engage in activities that lead to a lot of exposure to UV light, wind, or debris, you both need to be cool, put on some shades, and protect the vision you've got, whatever it is!

The Retina

Finally—we are now going to "focus" on the retina! This is where the anatomical differences in the eyes of humans and dogs are the greatest—and this is where everyone's favorite question will be answered—do dogs see color? The answer is yes—just not the same way we do.

First, some of the retinal differences between humans and dogs that have an impact on visual acuity: as mentioned previously, the retinas in both humans and dogs contain photoreceptors called cones and rods, but the type, quantity, and distribution of the cones and the rods differ greatly between humans and dogs. Cones, as you may remember, respond to color, and different types of cones respond specifically to certain colors of light, whereas rods respond best to white light. Humans have many more rods than cones—we have 120 million rods and six to seven million cones. But we make the most of our cones by concentrating them in the center of the retina, in the macula, and then concentrate them even further by having *only* cones in the tiny depression in the macula known as the fovea. This is the area where images are focused on the retina and where our vision is the sharpest.

In dogs, about 10 percent of their photoreceptors are cones, but the distribution in the retina is different than that of humans: the central 25 percent of the canine retina is composed of rods. In dogs, there is an oval area called the *area centralis* that is analogous to the human macula—the area where the density of rods and cones is highest. However, in contrast to humans, who have a cone-packed fovea in the center of the macula, where the vision is sharpest, dogs have a side-to-side stripe, which becomes wider on the side of the eye that is toward the side of the head, called the *visual streak* in which the density of rods is the highest and the visual acuity is best. The visual streak is present in other mammals as well, and is thought to aid in scanning the horizon, as it is roughly parallel to it. The bulge on the outside portion of the visual streak is thought to improve binocular vision, which can be limited by eye position, as mentioned earlier. There is some variation in the size of the visual streak among different breeds of dogs, and this may relate to the breed's purpose; dogs that were traditionally bred to hunt by sight, such as Greyhounds and Whippets, would need to be good at scanning the horizon, compared to those that hunt by scent, such as Blood Hounds and Beagles. These days, however, since many dogs are being bred for their appearance more than for their abilities, there is variation even within breeds in the size of the visual streak. That being said, little research has been done to determine whether or not this translates into better or worse vision within those different breeds.

Another interesting difference between the human retina and the dog retina is that, in dogs, the portion of the retina toward the feet, the inferior portion, has an even lower cone density than the rest of the retina. This area has, therefore, the very lowest visual acuity. This means that objects high in the field of vision are not seen very well, since, as you will recall, a visual image is projected upside-down on the retina. Since dogs have had very few airborne predators to worry about, this makes sense from an evolutionary standpoint. Remember this next time you toss something high in the air for your dog to catch—if your dog is not paying attention, it may just bounce off his head! That is, unless you do this in dim light—dogs have great sensitivity to motion, in general, as do humans, but dogs are especially tuned to motion in dim light. One study of dogs showed that they could recognize certain objects from a greater distance, as long as they were moving, but failed to recognize them at a closer distance, if they remained still. Motion detection in dogs is especially acute in the periphery of their visual fields, due to the higher rod density there compared to humans.

Second, humans and dogs have great differences in their respective sensitivities to light. As explained earlier, dogs have larger corneas than humans and pupils that tend to stay wider; these features allow more light to enter the eye of a dog than that of a human. Also, dogs have more rods than cones in the central part of their retinas, compared to humans, who have more cones than rods in a similar location, and, as a consequence, dogs have better visual acuity in dim light. However, there is another important adaptation to dim light that dogs possess that humans do not: once that extra light is inside the eyeball of a dog, it gets bounced around by a reflective coating in the superior (toward the top of the head) part of the retina called the *tapetum lucidum*. This beautiful, iridescent greenish coating is why most dogs' eyes look green when caught in flashlights or headlights at night. It gives the light that has already hit the retina a second chance to stimulate the photoreceptors and is an adaptation common in nocturnal animals. In cats, it is estimated that their eyes reflect about 130 times more light than human eyes, and, despite some anatomic differences, canine eyes are probably not much less reflective.

There is also an interesting variation in the location of the most reflective coating in the retina; the superior part of the retina receives light from the darker ground and the most reflective portion of the tapetum is located there, thus maximizing that light, while the light from the brighter sky is received in the inferior portion of the retina, and is less reflective.

Here's something else that I find fascinating—the tapetum may shift some of the reflected light to be closer to the wavelengths that stimulate rods, thus brightening a blue-black night sky, and increasing contrast between the sky and darker objects, such as predators, silhouetted against it. The only downside to these adaptations may be that the extra light allowed in and reflected around decreases the sharpness of the image focused on the retina. Then again, the fine facial details of a large, swiftly moving night predator are much less important to dogs than just detecting and avoiding the predator altogether, so trading night vision for sharp vision has not proved to be a bad deal for dogs!

And now, finally, color perception: remember that the perception of color is achieved by a complex process that starts with the stimulation of the photoreceptor cells in the retina and ends in the visual cortex and other areas of the brain, cones being the photoreceptors that respond to colored light. Color vision is the ability to distinguish objects based on the wavelengths (measured in nanometers [nm]) of the light they reflect. Colors are often grouped into seven general categories based on their wavelengths; from long (700 nm) to short (390 nm) wavelengths, they are red, orange, yellow, blue, indigo, and violet. Within each of these colors are millions of shades or hues, and mixing the pure colors together creates millions more colors.

Humans have three types of cones that respond to red, green, and blue light; dogs only have two types of cones that respond to violet and yellow-green light. Humans, because they have three kinds of retinal cones, can distinguish between very slight differences in the wavelengths of the reflected light—as little as one nm! As a species, humans can distinguish up to ten million colors, but the perception of colors can vary from one human to the next and can be influenced by age, experience, and even culture.

Dogs have two types of retinal cones—one is most sensitive to violet wavelengths (429–435 nm) and another with is most sensitive to yellow-green light (around 555 nm). It is not known whether dogs perceive these two colors in the same way that people do—after all, we can't even truly know exactly how individual members of our own species perceive color! That being said, some assumptions will be made here, based on what is known: the colors that dogs can see may be divided into two hues—one is in the wavelength range of 430–475 nm, and, whereas people see color in this range as violet to blue-violet, dogs probably see color in this range as blue; the other is in the 500–620 nm range, where humans see greenish-yellow, yellow, and red, but dogs probably only see yellow. For dogs, there is a narrow band within the

475–485 nm wavelength range, which would be blue-green for humans, but is without color for a dog and is seen as shades of white or gray. This is called that *spectral neutral point* and, in humans, this neutral point is in a greener area of the spectrum, at 505 nm. For humans, who have more cones in general, colors are seen as more saturated—that is to say, stronger and brighter—than they are by dogs, although colors at the two extremes of the visual spectrum, yellow and blue, are probably seen as more saturated by dogs than the middle portion.

Although dogs are often said to see color as do people with blue-green color-blindness (these are people that have inherited abnormalities in the function of the cones that respond to red and green areas of the visual spectrum), this is not really accurate, since dogs, with fewer cones, perceive colors in a less saturated way than humans. In addition, the difference between dogs and humans (including color-blind humans) in the location of the spectral neutral point, where there is no color, makes another difference in how color is perceived by dogs and humans with red-green color blindness. One more thing—despite the dogs' decreased ability to see colors, except in desaturated shades of blue, yellow, gray, and white, they have been reported to differentiate between closely related shades of gray that are not distinguishable by the human eye. This most likely helps in visual discrimination in very low lighting conditions.

One more thing—a very recent, absolutely fascinating discovery! Most dog lovers have seen either the older or newer version of the movie *Homeward Bound*—in which three lost pets (two dogs and one cat) become separated from their family and make their way home over many, many miles. The Internet is full of similarly miraculous stories—well, there may actually be some truth to those stories, and the reason may lie in the rods in the canine retina. Scientists have known for years that there are a group of light-sensitive molecules, called *cryptochromes*, that are found in bacteria, plants, birds, insects, reptiles, and fish, which enable them to sense magnetic fields. In addition to regulating of circadian rhythms, these molecules aid in the perception of direction, altitude, and location. It will come as no great surprise that we directionally impaired humans lack this molecule—but it has recently been found in the cones of dogs.[1] It's not clear yet how dogs might use this "sixth sense"—but it does make one wonder what else our dogs "see" that we can't.

How can we use this knowledge about color perception in dogs? Since dogs see yellow and blue the best of all the colors, try to choose toys that are these colors—especially those toys that are the strongest, most saturated versions of those colors. Guess what the most popular toy color is? Red—and only because this is a color we humans see well, and our eyes, and brains, will be stimulated to buy red toys. Of course, there is nothing wrong with red toys for dogs, since they probably see red as a slightly brighter shade of yellow. But some toys may be more simulating and fun for your dog if you pay attention to their color.

For example, let's say you usually play ball with your dog in a green, grassy field. The green grass probably looks brownish-yellow to your dog, and if you throw or roll a blue ball for your dog to fetch, he will probably see it better against the grass than a red, green, or yellow one. If you usually throw a Frisbee against a nice blue sky, using a black one may help your dog keep track of it better. If you hike with your dog off-leash, wear some clothing that he can see well against the surrounding environment, such as deep, bright blue, white, or black—the orange vests that people usually use to avoid being accidentally shot by hunters work well for that purpose since humans can see the difference be-tween the green forest and the orange vest, but they won't help dogs spot their owners since the green forest and the orange vest will look pretty much the same.

Knowledge about the color perception of dogs is also helpful in training for certain tasks—dogs that are trained to guide the visually impaired cannot distinguish red and green stoplights, but need to learn how to interpret the lights by the position, not the color, of the lights. For other tasks, dogs may not be able to be trained to choose between yellow, orange, green, or red objects based on their color, but changes in the brightness may help give dogs a way to distinguish them from each other. For agility training, when dogs compete as they jump over fences, run along balance beams or go through tunnels, the choice of equipment color is very important. Equipment that is blue, yellow, or white and that has contrast with the color of the ground underneath is best for the competitors—imagine how much harder it would be to jump over hurdles accurately if the hurdles, the ground underneath, and the background around them were all about the same color of gray. Attention to color, as seen through the eyes of your dog, will also come in handy as your dog ages and color perception, as well as other aspects of vision, change. More about that later.

Here is one last intriguing difference in human and canine vision and visual perception: *flicker fusion*. This is defined as the frequency at which an intermittent light stimulus appears to be continuous to the average human viewer and, not coincidentally, is the number of individual photos, or frames, per second that are needed to create the perception of smooth movement on TV. Too few frames per second will make the movement on the video appear jerky to humans—think of the way old movies, shot in the very early days of cinematography, look to us now. For humans, the flicker fusion rate is sixty frames per second. For dogs, it is seventy to eighty frames per second. It appears that the flicker fusion rate is roughly correlated, among different species, with how fast that species moves through their environment, because it is a measurement of how often the retina can update the image projected on it. Falcons, for example, can fly at speeds up to 242 mph and have a flicker fusion of more than one hundred frames per second! This is why your dog—and, I guess, your falcon—do not watch TV. Dogs may appear to watch TV—they may attend to individual images, or key into the jerky movement, since they are programmed to detect movement anyway, but they are probably paying more attention to the sound than anything else. Not being able to watch TV is not such a bad thing—maybe humans should *all* see like our dog and *not* be able to watch TV—we'd all get more exercise.

Now that you are an expert in dog vision and visual perception, how do you put all this information together to better understand your dog? Well, you will have to put on some caninomorphic spectacles and use some imagination! Plus you can go to the website howtoageproofyourdog.com for images and videos of how the world looks through your dog's eyes.

First, look around your home—note the colors of the furniture, the pillows, the accessories versus those of the floor or floor coverings. Subtract all that is red or green, and subtract the brightness of the colors. Notice, in your imagination anyway, how the floor and all the furniture items kind of blend together—you can see that your environment doesn't look the same, doesn't *mean* the same, as seen through your dog's eyes. Take a plastic sandwich bag—one of the more substantial ones, and look through it—this blurs your vision just a little and very roughly approximates your dog's decreased visual acuity. Next, try this outside, on a dull, gray, rainy day; notice how the colors of your yard or your neighborhood lose their punch—that, minus any reds or greens, with blurred vision, is how the outside world looks to your dog. Imagine you can't see very well either close up *or* far away—how do you recognize someone? Well, not so well if you only use your sense of sight— unless that someone moves! How could you read someone's facial expression? It would be hard to see a furrowed brow or a frowning mouth—unless you pay attention, as dogs do, to the overall body language.

Another informative—and fun—caninomorphic exercise to do is this: measure the height, from the ground, of your dog's eyes, then take your smartphone or camera, and video what the world looks like from that height. Tilt it up slightly to see what the upper reaches of your dog's world looks like, both inside your home, with all the furniture around, and also outside in some tall grass or in some bushes. If you can, change the color filter to "mono" or "tonal" to remove the color— this isn't exactly how color looks to your dog, but it does help you realize how different everything looks—including you! From that height and angle, it would be even harder to read a facial expression, especially for the smaller dogs. Also, think of how hard it would be, if you were an older dog with neck or back arthritis, to bend your neck and raise your head to look up at your owner. This type of exercise will help you so much to understand some of the changes in the behavior of your dog as he gets older.

And one last exercise, take a walk at night with your dog. As you both stride along, mentally project the visual field you, as a human, have and then try to see how much better you can see things, in the dim light, with the periphery of your vision. Also, turn your head slightly right and left to get an idea of the things your dog can see while he is looking straight ahead. Overall, watch your dog while you walk to observe all the things he is alerted to, based on a head turn, or the prick of the ears, that you can't see. Some of this is due to his superior vision in dim light, his superior motion detection, his superior peripheral vision, his superior visual field—but much is due to his vastly superior senses of hearing and smell, which, luckily, are our next topics.

7

THE LAUDATORY AUDITORY

Congress is so strange. A man gets up to speak and says nothing, nobody listens and then everybody disagrees. —Will Rogers

The dog's sense of hearing is very acute in comparison to that of a human, even during sleep, and is, like the sense of sight, specialized to alert the dog as early and accurately as possible to the approach and location of predators. This is good for their survival as a species, and their domestication has allowed humans to benefit, and sometimes survive, because of that hyperacute hearing. There are times when I would love to hear as well as my dogs—but I would, perhaps, prefer to sleep through all the small sounds that they hear through the night.

The basic mechanics of hearing are quite similar between humans and dogs, but, to understand hearing, one must first understand *sound*: sounds are vibrations that travel through a medium, such as air or water, as waves. The waves are caused by the vibration of objects; when something vibrates in air, like a violin string or a vocal cord, it moves the air particles around it. Those air particles, in turn, move the air particles around them by either squeezing the molecules of the surrounding air (called *compression*) or by pulling those molecules apart (*rarefaction*). When a group of molecules is squeezed, the area that contains them has an increase in pressure, and when they are pulled apart, there is a decrease in pressure. The amount of fluctuation (measured in *decibels* or dB) determines how loud the sound is, whereas the speed (or *frequency*) at which it fluctuates determines the pitch (measured in *Hertz*, Hz, or *kilohertz*, kHz, which is a unit of 1,000 Hz). As sound waves travel through a medium, they lose energy to that medium and, therefore, a sound wave can only travel a limited distance. In general, low frequency waves travel farther than high frequency waves because they transfer less energy to the medium.

If one of those objects is a dog's ear (such as that shown in figure 7.1), the dog's eardrum (*tympanic membrane*) will vibrate as well. This vibration is then passed along, through the air-filled *middle* ear, to three attached bones (the *malleus, incus* and *stapes*), the last of which pushes on another membrane, the *oval window*, to transmit the vibrations to a snail-shell-shaped, fluid-filled, coiled structure called the *cochlea*, which is contained within a space in the skull called the *bony labyrinth*. Sound vibrations in the air, at that point, are converted into waves

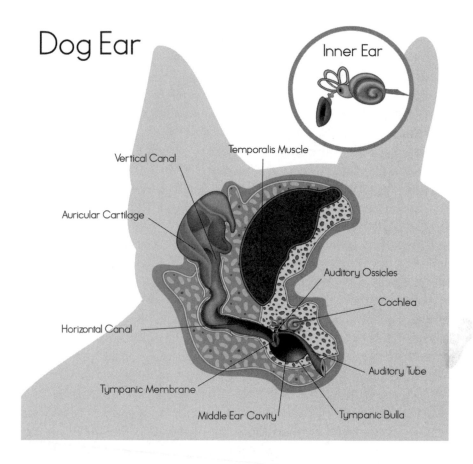

Dog Ear

Inner Ear

Temporalis Muscle

Vertical Canal

Auricular Cartilage

Auditory Ossicles

Cochlea

Horizontal Canal

Auditory Tube

Tympanic Membrane

Middle Ear Cavity

Tympanic Bulla

Figure 7.1.   Anatomy of the Canine Ear. Thinkstockphotos.com/*alexandragl1*.

within the fluid that is inside the cochlea. The tubular cochlea is coiled so it can have the maximum length possible in the tiny space of the inner ear.

The cochlea contains the *organ of Corti*, which has a membrane (the *basilar membrane*) running from end to end, splitting the tube into an upper and lower part. Hair cells (*cilia*) sit on top of the basilar membrane, and, projecting from each hair cell, are even smaller hair cells called *stereocilia*. As ripples travel through the fluid within the cochlea, the basilar membrane ripples as well, and the cilia, surfer-like, ride the wave, causing their stereocilia to bump into an overlying structure and bend. The bending causes tiny pores to open up—chemicals then flow into the pores and this creates an electrical signal. What is amazing about this is that each hair cell is tuned to a different frequency or pitch, and vibrates at specific locations along the cochlea in response to the different vibrations of the sound waves it receives. This means that a sound wave that is fluctuating rapidly will cause one group of cilia in one area along the length of the cochlea to vibrate, whereas a wave that is fluctuating slowly will have this effect in a different area of the cochlea.

Each cilia's individual nerve fiber transmits information about each individual sound frequency to the brain via the thirty thousand fibers of the *auditory nerve* (also called the *cochlear nerve*). The auditory nerve is one of the two branches of the *vestibulocochlear nerve* and sends the sound information to the brainstem; this information is then processed by various regions of the brain before it gets to the *superior temporal gyrus*, or auditory cortex, located on both sides of the brain. Within the auditory cortex, nerves are grouped together which respond to similar tones, but there are also "specialist" nerves that respond to different combinations and durations of tones, and some of these specialists combine that information to help the listener recognize words or music. Auditory information is processed in various regions of both halves of the auditory cortex, but the auditory cortex of the left side of the brain is, for humans and dogs, the area that allows us both to perceive certain sounds as speech. If this area is damaged, the listener may hear sounds created by another person, but not be able to process it in a way that allows the listener to understand them.

The structures of both the human and canine ear do more than just create the sense of hearing: the bony labyrinth contains another structure called the *semicircular canal*—this is actually composed of three attached semicircular channels (the *semicircular* ducts), which are oriented at right angles to each other. These channels contain fluid as well as microscopic pebbles called *cristae*; when the head or body rotates or tilts, the fluid in each of the ducts sloshes around, and the cristae are tumbled about like pebbles on a beach. There are two structures (the *utricle* and *saccule*) adjacent to the semicircular ducts, which are lined with cilia and are stimulated by the fluid and pebble motion. The way the fluid and pebbles move are a reflection of how the head and body are moving in space. This information is transmitted by the cilia to the second branch of the vestibulocochlear nerve, the *vestibular nerve*, and then on to the brain—and this is what the "sense of balance" is.

But how does sound reach the tympanic membrane in the first place? It is captured by the outer part of our ear (called the *pinna*) and then travels through the external ear canal, which is a tubular structure that, in dogs, has a vertical component and then bends to travel through the skull horizontally. In humans, the ear canal only has the horizontal component. In both humans and dogs, the skin lining the ear canal contains hair follicles and glands that produce wax to trap foreign material, such as dust, but the external ear canals of dogs are longer than those of humans and have more hair follicles and wax-producing glands.

The pinna's structure not only helps funnel sound to the tubular outer ear canal that leads to the tympanic membrane, it also helps the listener localize sounds. Pinnae are full of curves and crevices—sound waves that reach the pinnae will bounce off the curves and crevices of each ear differently, depending on the direction from which they came. The reflection of the vibrations alters the pattern of a sound wave, and our brains can recognize specific patterns that indicate if the sound originates in front, behind, below, or above the listener. In addition, the pinnae are located, in humans and dogs, toward the sides of the head. This allows the brain to determine the horizontal position of a sound by comparing the difference in the information coming from each ear. Humans have ears that are fairly uniformly shaped within our species— they are on the sides of our heads but are tipped slightly forward, and, party tricks aside, they are immobile. This allows humans to hear sounds in front of them better than those behind them.

The size, location, shape, and mobility of the pinnae are one of the major differences between human and canine hearing. Although there are significant breed variations, dogs have large pinnae that capture more sound than the pinnae of humans—to simulate how much better your dog can hear because of this, try cupping your hands around each of your pinnae to create a large surface area, and also try to vary the amount that you close your hand to experience how that alters the sound.

Depending on the breed of the dog, the pinnae are either erect or loosely folded down, and it would seem logical that those dogs with erect ears would hear better than those with floppy ears—but this has been shown not to be true, probably because floppy-eared dogs can move muscles to "prick up" their ears and this moves the floppy ends of the pinnae away from the outer part of the canals. Dogs have fifteen different muscles that can move their ears in many different directions, and they can also move one ear at a time, to capture the initial sound, after which they rotate both ears and their head to capture the maximum amount of sound. Studies have shown that dogs can localize a sound within an amazing 0.06 seconds! There are also some variations between breeds in the structure of the external ear canals—some breeds, like poodles, grow lots of hair in the ear canal, while others, like Boxers, have less, and this does not seem to impact the hearing either.

What *can* impact the hearing, however, is excessive wax or debris in the outer ear canal, since these are dense enough to dampen the conduction of the sound waves on their way to the tympanic membrane—and certain breeds of dogs have more wax-producing glands in their ear canals (called *ceruminous glands*) than others (and their owners can help them hear better by cleaning their ears regularly).

Despite these differences, the larger canine pinna provides a very effective funnel to direct sound toward the middle and inner ear, and this allows dogs to hear sounds from a much greater distance than humans—a sound that a human can only hear from one hundred yards away can be detected by a dog from a quarter of a mile away! All of this makes sense given the need for dogs to quickly and accurately localize predators in order to survive—and, luckily we humans have our dogs to localize *our* predators, since we aren't all that good at it!

So that's the outside story on the difference between dog and human hearing—and here's the inside story: dogs hear a much larger range of sound frequencies than humans. Their coiled cochleas are longer and coiled more tightly than ours, and there are, therefore, more stereocilia that are tuned to more frequencies. However, one important thing to note here is how difficult it is to actually measure how well dogs hear.

In humans, hearing acuity is usually measured when the human undergoing testing (usually while in a sound booth with earphones on) indicates that a sound that is being played in one ear has been heard. Since dogs have trouble reliably doing this, their hearing can be tested by measuring their brain's response to sounds using a Brain-Evoked Auditory Response (BAER) test, but this gives us limited real-world information. This makes the determination of the frequencies and intensities of the sounds that dogs, and other nonhuman species, can hear problematic—as is the determination of the canine sensitivity to sound. Sound sensitivity is a measurement of the frequencies that can be heard at various intensities, and except for profoundly deaf dogs, most frequencies can be detected if the sounds are produced loudly enough. The range of frequencies that dogs can hear has thus varied from study to study, but is generally accepted to be (from low to high frequency) between 67 Hz to 45 kHz, while humans hear in the range of 64 Hz to 23 kHz. This means that dogs can hear higher-pitched sounds than humans can, although we both have about the same low-pitch hearing limit. The reason for this difference is most likely due to the need of dogs, as a species, to tune in to the sounds of prey, especially those that are young or injured, as these are the ones that emit higher-pitched sounds. Puppies also emit high-frequency sounds, and the ability of mothers to hear those sounds is obviously helpful to puppy survival.

Humans don't hear as large a range of sounds as dogs do, but what we do hear is important to our species—we are specialized to hear in the frequency range used by human speech, and the human brain has the ability to use the order and combination of the words to create meaning. Studies have shown that dogs have a similar lateralization of these brain responses. In a 2012 study, researchers measured dogs' attention to speech or intonation. Dogs were led between two speakers and exposed to ten different types of speech or intonation, with use of a synthesizer. The human speech was altered and sometimes the dogs only heard emotional content and, at other times, dogs were exposed to words without any intonation. Results showed that dogs turned their heads to the left when sounds contained no words but had a positive intonation, indicating right hemispheric processing, and that they turned their heads to the right when familiar verbal commands in their own human's language were played, but not when the commands were in a foreign language—this indicated left hemispheric specialization.

This study demonstrated that dogs attend to both the speech and emotional content of human vocalizations. It also indicates that they process speech, meaning, and emotional content in a manner similar to humans. This finding was backed up by another study, published in 2014,[1] on the brain response to voice by both humans and dogs. It used a functional MRI (fMRI)—this is a way of creating an image of brain activity by detecting associated changes in blood flow within the brain. Since nerves need oxygen to function, and oxygen is carried by blood, the nerves that are most active will have greater blood flow. This type of imaging has been especially useful in certain types of research and in the diagnosis of some medical conditions since it does not require a response by the subject—just cooperation. This is why it is not used much in veterinary medicine because, in order to work, the patient must be awake and lie perfectly still—and most dogs will not lie perfectly still in a noisy MRI machine—except dogs that have been highly trained to do so, like those in this study.

This study was the first one to prove anatomically that dogs have areas in their brains that are analogous to those of humans in terms of location and activation during exposure to the same human vocalizations, dog vocalizations, nonvocal environmental sounds, and silence. Response to emotion was evaluated also, with the vocalizations ranging from highly positive to highly negative, and included whining and crying, barking and laughing. The greatest activity in the humans' brains was triggered by human voices, whereas the greatest activity in the dogs' brains was elicited by dog vocalizations. The results proved that specific areas in the canine brain are indeed devoted to making sense of vocalizations, and that are attuned to their emotional content. Other studies have proven that dogs can categorize sounds—they demonstrate recognition that a male voice goes along with a picture of a man, by looking longer at a picture of a man than at a picture of a woman when a male voice is played, and will gaze at a photo of a small dog longer than that of a large dog when listening to a high-pitched bark.

The frequency of the sounds we humans emit as speech ranges between 85 Hz and 255 Hz—vowels and some consonants ("z," "v," "m," "n," "d," "b") have low frequencies while other consonants ("s," "f," "th") have high frequencies. Babies emit sounds that are around 500 Hz, while children's speech ranges from 250–400 Hz, adult females tend to speak at around 200 Hz (range 165 to 255 Hz) and adult males around 125 Hz (range 85 to 180 Hz). This is for sounds emitted in a speaking voice—sound emitted by singing, at the same loudness or dB level, can go much higher. Note this range—as mentioned earlier, dogs hear well in the range of 67 Hz to 45 kHz, and this overlap of the hearing of dogs with the range of sounds that humans emit as speech is significant, since dogs, in the past, were likely selected for their ability to hear, and, to some extent, understand what their human companions were saying. This was important then—and is important for you to be aware of now—and especially in the future, as your dog ages and loses some portions of his hearing range. More about that later.

Low-pitched sounds, such as a male voice, can travel better than high-pitched sounds, such as a female voice. A female speaker who wants to give a command to a dog from a distance, as would be true for herding, needs to raise the loudness level of her voice higher than would a man in order for the dog to hear the command. That being said, dogs hear high pitches very well, and a command that is sung from a distance might be heard even better, since the singing voice can raise the pitch of vocalizations by up to four octaves! Studies have shown that dogs can discriminate between the vowel sounds imbedded in human speech, which are produced at a low frequency, and since vowel sounds are crucial in identifying individual words, this is a crucial point in the question of whether dogs understand language. Dogs use phonetic information in order to identify a wide variety of individual words, as demonstrated by a study in 2005,[2] which took some of the sounds out of commands that the test dogs had previously learned; this, not surprisingly, led to a decrease in the number of correct responses.

Studies have also shown that dogs clearly understand how the sounds humans make go together to make words with certain meanings. But can dogs understand what those words mean if they are put together in a different way to convey a different meaning? Understanding individual words, after all, is not the same as understanding language. To know the answer to this question, one must find dogs that can consistently demonstrate that they understand the meaning of a list of individual words, as well as a list of short combinations of words, and then test those dogs' understanding of the words when they have been combined in a different way.

Several studies have been done on dogs that have been taught to fetch certain toys when identified by their individual names.[3] One famous Border Collie, Rico, learned the names of two hundred different toys, and repeatedly demonstrated that he knew the names by retrieving the correct item (when asked by his owner to "fetch X") from a pile of ten toys located in a different room. He also learned new names for new items quickly—usually after only one presentation of the object while its name was said by the owner! Although this proved that Rico had an amazing ability to learn individual word labels, and that he understood he was supposed to fetch the items that matched the label, it did not prove that he knew that the word "fetch" carried a meaning separate from the word ("X") that followed it.

Another study, using a dog named Chaser (also a Border Collie) was designed to prove this point. Chaser, amazingly, was taught the names of over one thousand objects (such as "ball" and "stick"), as well as many different commands (such as "take" or "paw") telling what to do with the objects, and then the commands and the objects were mixed up to see if Chaser could perform the right task with the right object. Chaser passed this test by responding correctly to new combinations of objects and actions (such as "take ball" versus "paw ball"). In another study, a dog named Sophia did even better by responding correctly to novel combinations of objects and actions when the order was reversed, such as "stick fetch" versus "stick point." Further studies with Chaser showed that she was aware of word order and simple grammatical rules—she was taught to respond to sentences including three elements of grammar: a preposition, a verb, and a direct object (such as "to ball take Frisbee"), and she responded correctly when the object labels were reversed.

These studies showed that at least these dogs understood which words referred to objects and which to action—but does that mean dogs understand the symbolic nature of words—that is, do they just associate the word and object together, or do they understand that a certain word could refer to an absent object? Another study tested the ability of dogs to associate symbols—visual replicas—with objects. Rico was again used for this study, plus some other less famous Border Collies, and they were simply, silently, shown a replica, either a full-size drawing, a miniature drawing, or a photograph of the object they were to fetch from another room—and they did it! This demonstrates not only that these dogs understand symbols—verbal, visual, and probably more—but that they also understand what humans want, are ripe to learn new ways to work with us, and are always learning from us. One study even showed that dogs can learn the names of new objects just by hearing two people speaking about them repeatedly before asking the dog to retrieve it, and this proves that our close canine companions are primed to learn from us even when we don't try to train them.

Our complex vocal apparatus allows us to say a lot to our dogs, and most of us talk a lot to our dogs—and often using the high-pitched voice that adults use to speak to young children. This is probably no accident—dogs seem to respond well to this type of vocalization, and reward their owners by giving all the correct signals that they are enjoying it—maybe the fact that dogs hear so well at those higher frequencies has something to do with that. Although your dog's less complex vocal apparatus keeps him from talking back to you, at least in words, remember how great his hearing is. Whether your dog is actually responding on the left side of his brain to the content of your speech, and perceiving the language of your vocalizations, or responding on the right side of his brain, to the emotional content of your speech, or both, he is a member of a species that has been selected to understand your communications. When there is one species that can say a lot, and another that can hear a lot, a great partnership can form!

Your new knowledge about the auditory capabilities of your canine companion can help you choose your words well—or at least your tone and volume. Remember that dogs hear and respond to higher vocal frequencies, that different components of speech (vowels, consonants) have different frequencies, that dogs can hear at lower decibel levels, and that low tones travel further than high tones. Remember also that communication seems to be a basic need of both the *homo sapiens* and *canis familiaris* species—so take advantage of that as you go through your daily lives together and talk to your dog often. He not only hears, but perceives, more than you could ever say.

8

SMELL SCENTRAL

Smell is a potent wizard that transports you across thousands of miles and all the years you have lived. —Helen Keller

When I was in anatomy class during my first year of veterinary school, I saw the canine brain for the first time. What amazed me was that the part of the brain that corresponded with the perception of smell appeared much larger than other parts of the brain and even had an elongated portion that extended, literally, to the back of the nose itself, as if all the scent molecules funneled in that direction by the nose were to go directly to the brain. This, of course, is not actually true—there are lots of things that happen to those scent molecules before the dogs perceive them, but the size of that portion of the canine brain does demonstrate the importance of this particular sense to their species. The area of the canine brain that is devoted to the analysis of smells, the olfactory lobe, is forty times bigger than the analogous area in the human brain. Although there are some rare human individuals, called "super smellers" (mostly employed by perfume manufacturers or wine makers), who can, through rigorous training and years of experience, identify hundreds or thousands of different odors, they can't even come close to your own dog's inborn, untrained sense of smell.

Humans have 350 genes that are responsible for odor perception—dogs have 971. Humans have six million smell, or olfactory, receptors in their noses—dogs have, depending on the breed, up to three hundred million! Why do dogs have so many olfactory receptors? Partly because a keen sense of smell aids in the detection of prey and predator and, therefore, increases survival of their species, and partly because dogs use their sense of smell in a social way—to identify friends, foes, family members, and willing mates, as well as their emotional state and health status.

Historically, dogs were used and selected by hunting humans for the ability to track prey by their sense of smell, and, over the years, scent hounds such as Beagles, Basset Hounds, and Bloodhounds were selected to became the "super smellers" of the canine species—studies have shown that these dog breeds actually have more smell receptors in their noses than other breeds. More recently, dogs—even members of breeds not known to be "super smellers"—are being used for a variety of olfactory tasks. One study even showed Pugs far outperforming German Shepherds in scent detection! Governmental agencies use dogs, usually big ones such as Labrador Retrievers, Golden Retriever, German Shepherds, Belgian Malinois, and mixed-breed dogs, to detect drugs and agricultural contraband, to search for lost individuals or homicide victims. U.S. Customs and Border Patrol has more than eight hundred canine teams that work with the U.S. Department of Homeland Security to combat terrorist threats, find illegal narcotics, and detect unreported currency, concealed humans, and prohibited fruits, plants, or meats in baggage. Some dogs are even being trained to detect low blood sugar in diabetic humans, to warn of an imminent seizure in people with epilepsy, and to find prostate or breast cancer. The number of ways humans exploit this canine superpower seems to be ever growing, as is our understanding of what happens between smell and brain cell.

Here is what we know so far: First, what triggers the sense of smell? The basic unit of an odor is a molecule of a volatile chemical compound—that is, a compound that was once a solid which then turned into a gas and became suspended in air. Those odor molecules first encounter the cold, moist exterior portion (also called the "leather" or *nasal planum*) of the dog's nose, get stuck on the mucus layer on its surface and then dissolve to be carried to the interior of the nose by the mucus itself. Odor molecules can also be captured by sniffing—when a dog or human sniffs and forcefully draws air carrying odorant molecules into her nostrils, there are many folds and crevices within the nose that funnel the molecules to a specialized area in the roof of the nasal cavity. This small area (only a few centimeters wide) contains the *olfactory epithelium*, which is that specialized membrane that contains millions of *olfactory receptors*. Each olfactory receptor has a *cilia*, which is a hair-like projection that increases the surface area of the receptor and increases the chance that it will interact with an odorant molecule. Each cilia is surrounded by moisture-secreting tissue. The olfactory epithelium is, therefore, moist, and the odorant molecules stick to it, dissolve, and then bind with the olfactory receptor proteins. This initiates a cascade of chemical and electrical events that lead to the firing of each receptor's individual *olfactory neuron*, or nerve cell. The millions of olfactory neurons from each side of the nose together make up the *olfactory nerves*, also called Cranial Nerve 1. They each run through tiny holes in a bone, called the *cribriform plate*, which is located in the back of the nasal passages and is the only thing separating the nose from the brain. The olfactory neurons from each side of the nose then are clustered together into the *olfactory bulbs*, then into the *olfactory tracts* and these terminate in the *olfactory lobes* of the *cerebral cortex* of the brain.

Although humans and dogs possess an impressive number of olfactory receptors, there are many, many more odor molecules in the world than there are receptors in the nose. How can animals detect and then discriminate between so many odors?

To begin with, each dissolved odor molecule typically activates several olfactory receptors, depending on the number of molecules of a certain odorant that are present, and each receptor can detect several related odorants. Which olfactory receptors are activated and the intensity of the activation help to create an "odorant pattern" unique to that odor, which the brain ultimately perceives as a specific odor. The task of processing odors continues in the olfactory bulb—this area has three functions: the discrimination between odors, the enhancement of the sensitivity of odor detection, and the rejection of background odors to enhance the transmission of certain odors. The odors are then sorted out further in various parts of the olfactory cortex.

One area, the *anterior olfactory* cortex, detects and stores correlations between olfactory features, and forms olfactory representations, or *gestalts*, of particular odorants and odorant mixtures. Another area, the *piriform cortex*, processes the gestalts themselves and, starts to categorize them based on information stored in other parts of the brain about behavior and context. The *periamygdaloid cortex* participates in emotional processing of olfactory stimuli and starts to encode the information into memory, and the *entorhinal cortex* functions as a hub for memory and navigation. All of this information ultimately is relayed to the orbitofrontal cortex which interprets the olfactory signal. This, by the way, is the area of the brain that is involved in the integration of *all* sensory stimuli with prior experiences.

The superiority of the canine sense of smell, in comparison to that of humans, thus starts with the fact that dogs have more olfactory receptors per square inch of olfactory epithelium, which itself encompasses sixty times more square inches of odor-gathering intranasal surface area, and ends with the fact that their olfactory lobes are four times bigger than that of humans, accounting for one-eighth of the dog's total brain volume—but that is not even close to the complete story. The way the odor molecules get to the receptors in the first place tells the rest of the tale: in humans, the air we breathe is the air we smell—that is, we both breathe and smell through our noses. In dogs, a fold of tissue just inside each of their nostrils splits the air they sniff into two flow paths— one for smelling and one for breathing. When humans inhale through our noses, all the air is directed to the olfactory epithelium; when dogs

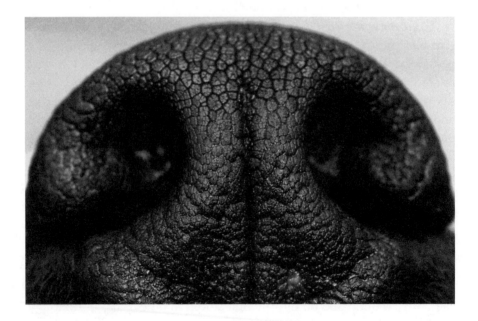

Figure 8.1.   The Amazing Canine Nose. Thinkstockphotos.com/*nemoris*.

inhale through their noses, about 12 percent of that air is directed to a recessed chamber, which is lined with olfactory epithelium, in the back of the nose, while 88 percent of the air goes down the throat to the lungs.

This chamber has labyrinthine scrolls of tissue, called the *nasal turbinates*, that are lined with millions of olfactory receptors, and these tissues sort out the different odor molecules based on their chemical properties and immediately start the process of odor analysis. What happens to the air after it has delivered its olfactory payload? In humans, the air just goes out the same way it came in, and that exhaled air keeps new odor molecules from entering until the next sniff. In dogs, the air goes out through slits in the sides of the nostrils, which you can see in figure 8.1. This does two important things: the swirling air pattern which is created by the air forced through the side-slits actually helps bring new odor molecules to the front of the nose, and it allows dogs to sniff almost continuously. Air can't enter the slits, but goes into each nostril in a fairly tight stream, and this allows dogs to detect into which nostril a certain odorant has entered. This, along with the ability of dogs to move each nostril independently, helps dogs locate the source of the odor.

The ability to sniff maximizes the detection of odors because the odor molecules that enter the olfactory chamber from one sniff and aren't recognized immediately, can stick around and accumulate to intensify the interaction with the olfactory epithelium. According to Resi Garritsen and Ruud Haak in their book *K9 Scent Training*, a dog at rest typically breathes in and out fifteen times per minute, and, while walking, breathes at a rate of thirty-one times per minute. However, when actively sniffing, a dog's breathing rate goes up to 140–200 times per minute. Scent detection dogs and hunting dogs use a technique called air scenting which uses one very long inhalation, followed by an exhalation through the mouth. This breathing pattern transfers a huge number of scent molecules to the olfactory epithelium. A study done in Norway showed that a hunting dog holding her head up into the wind in search of game sniffed in a continuous stream of air for up to forty seconds, while simultaneously inhaling and exhaling from her lungs thirty times. You have probably seen your own dog doing something like that while sticking her nose out the window or putting up what we, in our house, call "the nose periscope"—when dogs try to sniff out what delectable item is above their reach on the kitchen counter. And just think how often your dog sniffs every day!

How do dogs keep from being overwhelmed and confused by that continuous barrage of odors, given the billions of odor molecules he takes in with every sniff, snort, and snuffle? The brain, in general, tends to ignore continuous stimuli and notices differences and changes—this process is called *habituation*. After continuous exposure to an odor, the perception of it fades quickly, but recovers rapidly after that odor is removed. When odorants are mixed, the brain will block out the continuous odorants, although this can be affected by the strength of the odors in the mixture, which can change perception and classification of the odors. This process helps classify similar odors as well as adjust sensitivity to differences in complex stimuli. Since a single odor is typically recognized by multiple receptors, and different odors are recognized by combinations of receptors, the pattern of neuronal signals is what identifies a smell. Dogs are not only good at getting a lot of smell molecules in their noses, they are also good at understanding what those patterns mean—hence their increasing use in the detection of explosives and illicit drugs, the tracking of lost or fleeing humans, and the location of bodies after an explosion or natural disaster.

Working dogs use their noses in three different ways: tracking, trailing, and air sniffing. In tracking, the dog follows the scent of footprints on the ground and vegetation with his nose down—interestingly, the length of the tracking dog's ears may have a role in his skill in this task, since long ears dragging on the ground will kick odor molecules up into the air for the sniffing nose to capture! In trailing, dogs are following a scent suspended in the air—what they are following in either method is believed to be tiny bits of skin cells, covered by sweat and bacteria, which are lost from the human body at an astounding rate of five hundred million cells per minute. A study done in 2014 tested the existence of this human "fallout" by using German Shepherds that were trained in scent detection. These dogs were 100 percent correct in identifying specific individuals by an object above which they had held their hands at a distance of 3 cm, and confirmed that dogs can detect human scent trace without actual contact between humans and objects. Dogs seem to pay a *lot* of attention to the products of *apocrine glands* both in humans and their own species—these are specialized glands that, in humans, are located in the armpits and groin areas, and that, in dogs, are located on the entire body surface area. The odorants produced by these glands give the "sniffer" information about the age, gender, health status, and emotional state of the "sniffee." Some of these chemicals are present in high concentrations in tears, urine, sweat, and blood, as well as genital and anal area secretions—and those are of particularly intense (and, to a human "sniffee," embarrassing) interest to dogs.

In the case of tracking, what the dogs are following in the scent left behind by the part of the body that has the most sweat glands per square inch—which are the feet. The feet also have many *sebaceous glands*, which produce oils for our skin and hair, and this combination of sweat, fatty acids, cellular debris, and bacteria create a scent that will actually penetrate anything covering the feet (sock, insole, shoe, sole) to reach the underlying surface they have touched. This "foot fetish" can explain why so many people come home to find their dog has found and chewed their shoes—the shoes, after all, have the strongest scent of their favorite person, whom they have been missing, and brings them as close as possible—maybe "abscents" make the canine heart grow fonder?

Dogs are also being used to identify certain disease states in people—for example, I have a client who has a life-threatening allergic reaction to paprika and has an assistance dog trained specifically for that purpose who has undoubtedly saved her life many times. But paprika has a pretty strong smell—what about something more subtle? Dogs, even those that have not been trained to do so, can detect when their diabetic owner's blood sugar dips too low, even before the owner is aware of it, and have been able to alert their owners to eat something before that happens. This phenomenon seems to involve the dogs' ability to identify an olfactory change in some component (so far unidentified by human researchers) in their owner's perspiration as the blood sugar goes down.

You might be justified in thinking "It's all very well that a dog can detect this, but what do they do with that knowledge—what if the owner has already fainted or had a seizure from low blood sugar?" Well, Melody Jackson, a computer scientist at Georgia Tech has been working on that—she has developed wearable tech for service dogs, which allows them to pull a lever on their computerized vest triggers that an SOS with GPS coordinates, or another one that triggers an audio message asking for help after they have found another human. In addition, dogs, with some training, can reliably differentiate, via their sense of smell, urine samples of human patients with and without prostate cancer. There are many anecdotal reports of untrained dogs alerting their owners to the presence of breast cancer—this has led to research at Duke University on the use of dogs to screen for breast cancer, versus benign breast tumors, in the blood and breath of human patients, as well as at the University of California–Davis on the use of dogs to screen for throat cancer in human saliva. This is truly a sensory superpower! Impressed yet?

Now prepare to get even more impressed! You may have heard of "second sight," but have you heard of "second smell"? Probably not, since I just made it up. Nonetheless, it is an apt term here—*second sight* refers to the ability to perceive things that are not available to the senses, and I am using *second smell* to refer to the ability of dogs to perceive smells that are not available to our human senses. Many people (including me, until I went to vet school) are unaware that dogs have an additional, but very important, olfactory system for which there is no human parallel. This is the *vomeronasal organ* (also called Jacobson's organ) which consists of a pair of elongated, fluid-filled sacs that open into either the mouth or the nose, and is located above the roof of the mouth behind the upper front teeth (incisors). This area is specialized to detect *pheromones*—this is a term coined in the 1950s from the Greek *pherein*, meaning "to carry" and *hormone*, meaning "to excite," and literally means "carrier of excitement." These are volatile chemicals emitted by one member of a species that can affect the behavior and physiology of another member of the same species. These chemicals, which are not technically odorants or smells, are primarily messages about sex, changing hormonal levels, and mating readiness, and thus are, indeed, carriers of excitement, although they may also aid in communication about other aspects of social behavior.

The chemical constituents of pheromones start the pathway to the vomeronasal organs after sticking to the moist outer surface of the nose, where they then dissolve and travel as a liquid, via a pumping mechanism, to the olfactory receptors in the vomeronasal organs. This process is different than that for odorants, which must travel through the air before binding to the olfactory receptors. The olfactory receptors in the vomeronasal organs are also different than those in the main olfactory area of the nasal cavity in that they have no cilia, but do have little folds in their surface, called *microvilli*, to trap the liquefied molecules. Once binding occurs in the olfactory receptors, the olfactory neurons send the signals to an accessory olfactory bulb, dedicated to this area, and then on to the *hypothalamus*, the region of the brain which among other functions (including, not coincidentally, the production of hormones) is associated with sexual and social behaviors.

There is a characteristic dog behavior associated with activation of the vomeronasal organ—a dog will often push his tongue rapidly against the roof of his mouth, and then display some very quiet teeth chattering. This most often will occur after the dog sniffs or licks a spot of urine, but also after a male dog has detected the pheromone-filled secretions from a female dog in heat. Although perfume makers have been trying to develop a human sex pheromone for years, they have been unsuccessful—it is probably a futile task, since humans not only don't possess a functioning vomeronasal organ (we seem to only have a remnant), we don't even have an accessory olfactory bulb to transmit the signals to the brain. Perhaps it is best that way—humans have enough distractions already! However, there is some evidence that we can detect pheromones via our olfactory system, even without a vomeronasal organ, and research into this is ongoing—so ambitious perfume makers and hopeful singles can continue to dream.

So, how can we use this knowledge? There is no caninomorphic exercise to help you understand what it is like to have your dog's sense of smell, since humans lack both the necessary nasal apparatus and neural connections, but I guess we can use our new knowledge plus our creativity to imagine what our dogs are experiencing through their olfactory senses. For example, if dogs can smell something as subtle as lowering blood sugar through sweat, are they smelling our own state of mind through our sweat—our happiness, our depression, our stress, our fear? I think many dog owners would say their dogs do that all the time! Watch your dog's reaction to you as you go through different emotional states—does he not only react to it, but does he try to do something to change it? It's possible you already have an assistance dog without even knowing it!

You can also use your dog's sense of smell to keep him—and you—entertained, stimulated, and active. The sport of "nosework" is a competitive activity created to mimic the tasks that professional detection dogs perform. This sport involves competition between teams made up of one dog and one handler; the dogs must find a hidden target odor and then alert the handlers, after which the dogs are rewarded with food or a toy. One of the cool things about the sport of nosework is that dogs that are blind or have behavioral problems, such as aggression to dogs or humans, can participate since it appeals to every dog's sensory superpower and allows them to work alone and gain confidence.

Of course, you don't have to enter a competition or even a class to do nosework at home with your dog—in fact, you may already be doing it! Lots of my clients play "hide-and-seek" with their dogs—sometimes using treats and sometimes using their own bodies for their dogs to find. (I chuckled a little bit when one of my more straitlaced, elderly clients described her daily game of hide-and-seek and I then visualized all the contortions she had to have gotten into to hide from her little Teacup Poodle!) If you are playing hide-and-seek, your dog is, of course, following your scent trail. You can make this more challenging by using something (a treat or toy) that your dog really, *really* loves—and also has a strong scent, such as popcorn—and hiding it around your home. First, have your dog stay in one location, either in a stay position or restrained by someone else, then place the treat or popcorn around a corner and just slightly hidden so he's not just spotting it with his eyes. Let him loose, and let him find it—don't make it too challenging at first so that he won't get frustrated. You should encourage and praise him when he's close, or even point it out to him if he's having trouble at first.

Be sure to make it fun and enjoyable—but as your dog becomes more skilled at sniffing things out, make it more challenging by placing the object under or on furniture, under rugs, up on a windowsill. Make a big deal about the "find" and give a great reward—trust me, you will be rewarded, too! Praise him, pet him, and give the treat—by the way, two separate studies showed that, in one study, dogs preferred praise to treats, and, in the other study, they preferred petting to praise—personally, I think the best thing to do is pull out all the stops and use all three methods, thus appealing to the sense of hearing, the sense of taste as well as the sense of touch! But if your dog seems to enjoy the treat the most, you are about to understand why—but it isn't as simple as you might think.

9

TWO MORE SENSIBLE SENSES

TASTE

Taste is the common sense of genius. —Victor Hugo

Taste, in both humans and dogs, is really more about the nose than it is about the tongue. If you have ever had a bad cold that completely clogged your nose, you know how true that statement is. The anatomy of the tongue allows both species to detect certain flavors, which stimulates salivary glands to produce different types of fluids that are specialized to the types of food being consumed. The fluid's purpose is to dissolve chemicals in the food which, in turn, become volatile gases that go up from the back of the mouth right into the nose to stimulate the olfactory glands. This phenomenon is called *retronasal olfaction* ("retro" means "backward" in Latin) whereas what we usually think of as the act of smelling something—that is sniffing into the front of the nose—is called *orthonasal olfaction*. Tasting something, therefore, stimulates two separate neural pathways to the brainstem and then to the cerebral cortex, and this isn't always consciously processed—both taste and smell are influenced by instinctual species-specific nutritional needs as well as that individual's past experience, memories, and emotion. For dogs, with sixty times more smell receptors than humans, the sense of taste is strongly influenced by the sense of smell and is probably the reason that many dogs gulp down their food without even chewing it. Apparently, if it smells good, it will taste good, so no need to chew and savor it!

But if the nose is so important in the sense of taste, why bother with taste buds? Taste receptors in the tongue are really there for safety, not pleasure. Specific taste buds are tuned to detect different chemical groups—bitter and sour tastes are often associated with poisonous substances, and detecting those tastes early in the process of ingesting them, even before being conscious of them—allows the taster to spit them out before they can do any harm. We usually think of taste buds as being on the tongue, and they are indeed found within the bumps, or *papillae*, that are on the tongue's surface. Each papilla contains a pore, which are entered by dissolved chemical compounds from food in order to encounter clusters of taste receptors. However, many people don't realize that there are also taste buds located in other areas of the digestive tract—on the roof of the mouth, in the back of the mouth where it merges with the throat, inside the cheeks, in the upper esophagus, and in the intestine—but these taste buds are not connected to the nose or brain in the same way that the ones on the tongue are. The taste buds in the tongue transmit their gustatory information to the brain via the seventh, ninth, and tenth cranial nerves. The taste buds in the intestine are thought to trigger hormonal responses to salt and sugar, for example, or to stimulate evacuation, by vomiting or diarrhea, of potentially harmful substances.

Different species have different taste abilities and taste preferences, based on the niche they occupy in the world and the nutrients that they require for survival. Cats, for example, are strict carnivores and have no need to taste sweet flavors, which would be contained in carbohydrate-based foods. They have apparently evolved without the gene that encodes the "sweet" taste receptor. Humans are omnivores and need both meat-based foods and carbohydrates, as well as certain fats, vitamins, and minerals, to maintain healthy cellular function. Sugars, for example, have been evolutionarily important to us, and we will, unless our higher brain power takes over, eat too much of them, whether they be found in fruits, potatoes, or cupcakes. Salt is similarly important to us because it is not found in fruits and vegetables, so we need to seek it out in order to maintain an optimal fluid balance in our cells—but our desire for it sometimes outstrips our need.

It is apparently a matter of debate whether dogs are carnivores, like cats, or omnivores, like humans, and the jury is still out on that topic. It is clear that they, as descendants of the wolf species, started out as omnivores and maintain many digestive similarities to wolves, but, because dogs co-evolved with humans while that species evolved from a hunter-gatherer species to an agrarian one, they have also developed a few adaptive genetic changes in order to digest the food—usually the leftovers from their humans—that they were given. Dogs do have a higher meat requirement than humans—in the wild, 80 percent of their diet is meat. But, along with their humans, they, too, have developed a taste for sugars, although they do not have much drive to acquire additional salt, since the extra meat they consume already contains so much of it.

Dogs have 1,700 taste buds, while humans have four thousand, which, interestingly, is inversely proportional to each species' respective numbers of olfactory receptors. The sense of taste in both dogs and humans is present at birth and, in both species, can be influenced by the diet of the mother while she is pregnant, and the fetus's exposure to certain chemical compounds via the amniotic fluid. The sense of taste in both species takes time to develop fully after birth—for dogs, at least several weeks. The tastes that humans and dogs can detect appear to be the same—I say "appear" since dogs cannot report to us what they taste, and much research in taste perception in dogs has been through human observation of how fast or enthusiastically laboratory dogs eat certain test foods. The five basic tastes are: *sweet, salty, bitter, sour,* and *umami* (also called savory or meaty).

The arrangement of taste buds on the tongue of humans and dogs is also similar, although all areas of the tongue can respond to any flavor if it is in a high concentration. For humans, the area of the tongue most tuned to sweet tastes is in the front, whereas in dogs, it is toward the sides. For both species, the taste buds that are sensitive to sour and salty tastes are on the sides of the tongue, but, in dogs, they are further back, and the area that is sensitive to salty tastes is very small. The area of the tongue specialized for bitter is toward the very back of the tongue in both humans and dogs, while meaty tastes are best detected on the top of the tongue, especially toward the front.

Not surprisingly, the taste buds of dogs are specialized to detect amino acids, the basic building blocks of protein. They display a mild aversion to sour tastes, such as citrus, but a strong aversion to bitter tastes. This accounts for the use of citrus odors as deterrents for dogs, such as in citronella bark collars, and for the use in our clinic of the "bitter apple" solution we sometimes squirt on bandages to keep dogs from chewing them off—although this doesn't always work since the receptors for bitter are located at the back of the tongue, and a dog may have already torn off the bandage by the time he tastes it! Beware of mint-flavored dog treats, rinses, or toothpastes—humans associate that taste with good-smelling breath and cleanliness, but for dogs, mint falls in the bitter category, and they will react to them negatively after the first taste and will avoid that product forever.

Did you know that there is also a taste bud for "water"? Probably not, since humans don't have it. Dogs, like other carnivores (score one for those that say dogs are true carnivores) such as cats, have an area on the tips of their tongues that is specialized to respond to water, and becomes more sensitive to the water taste if they have eaten something salty or sweet. This may have been a mechanism that evolved to help drive carnivores to drink lots of water with their high-meat, and therefore high-salt, diet in order to keep an optimal fluid balance within their cells.

Dogs do prefer meat flavors over vegetable flavors, although they can become a victim of their own sensory superpower if an odor associated with meats is applied to vegetable products—a weakness discovered long ago by manufacturers of dry dog food. There is a whole industry devoted to the research and development of flavorants that are added to dog foods, and much of that information is proprietary—making the research about taste perception in dogs unavailable to the average person. Some studies on food preferences that are available to the public show that dogs prefer:

- beef to pork to lamb to chicken to horsemeat (used a lot in early canned dog foods in the early automobile era when horses were, sadly, being disposed of) to sweetened foods
- cooked meat to raw
- warm meat to cold
- wet or moist food to dry
- novel foods to familiar foods (for about three days, then the novel food becomes familiar)
- higher-fat foods to lower-fat foods
- sweet to meaty foods, if the sense of smell is impaired
- anything fed from the owner's hand to anything in a dish

These are useful points to know when you are choosing foods for your dog, or enticing him to eat if he is not feeling well. Warming food, adding water to food, and cooking food will all release volatile compounds, intensify the odor of the food and, therefore, its taste. However, studies have also shown that the flavor has to be as good as the smell's promise—even though they eat fast, dogs will slow down or stop eating a food that has little flavor even if it smells great, and will often not eat it the next time they encounter it. This illustrates that taste preferences are also influenced by experience, both positive and negative, showing that the brain is involved in the perception of taste.

Emotional associations with foods, the visual appearance of food, and preconceptions about foods seem to be very much more important in human taste perception than in canine taste perception. For example, people that taste wines of different prices rank a wine higher on taste if they know that wine is expensive, but, when the label is hidden, will often prefer the less expensive wine. Why is this important in a book about dogs? Because our human perceptions and biases about taste can also influence the choice of food for our dogs. Just like people who think the more expensive wine tastes the best, owners will often think that the most expensive dog food will taste the best to their dogs, or be the best nutritionally. Foods that are visually appealing to humans will often be perceived by humans as tasting the best to their dogs, when their dogs probably don't even see the food they are gulping down. The aroma of the food is what is most important to dogs, but the dog food manufacturers have to be careful about balancing that—what smells good to a dog will often not smell good to a human (think of the kinds of things that dogs like to roll in) and what is strong enough for a human to smell might be overpowering to a dog's stronger sense of smell.

Our human fads regarding diet are heavily influencing our food choices for our pets—there are vegetarian diets for cats, which, as a species, are strict carnivores and need actual meat. Veterinarians, like me, field questions almost every day about whether or not dogs should be on grain-free diets ever since the gluten-free trend started a few years ago. Raw diets are also popular, although, as mentioned previously, dogs, given the choice, actually prefer cooked meat. I mention all of this here so that you can be an informed buyer of your dog's food, and can see beyond the fads and ads—recommending certain foods is beyond the scope of this author and this book, but do discuss your dog's diet with your veterinarian. There is also a very useful website created by the World Small Animal Veterinary Association (wsava.org) with a downloadable pdf called: "The Savvy Dog Owner's Guide: Nutrition on the Internet" which has great tips on how to find good—and avoid bad—nutritional information. The website also has many links to other websites with reliable information about pet food, pet nutrition, raw food diets, home-cooked diets, obesity, and nutritional supplements. As with anything, education is the key to good choices for your dog.

TOUCH

Touch has a memory. —*John Keats*

The sense of touch is both basic and complicated, warns us of danger and assures us of love, is one of our first sensations, and, perhaps, one of our last. Also known as the *somatosensory system*, the sense of touch in humans and dogs is, in many ways, very similar in its physiology and in its importance to both of our species. It all starts at the receptor level, and many different types of receptors are found in many different locations in the body, specialized to detect specific sensations, such as temperature (*thermoreceptors*), light (*photoreceptors*), touch (*mechanoreceptors*), chemicals (*chemoreceptors*), pain (*nociceptors*), and the position of the body in space (*proprioceptors*). These are located in the skin, muscles, bones, joints, internal organs, and cardiovascular system.

Once the receptors detect an object, the information is transmitted via sensory nerves through tracts in the spinal cord to the brain, primarily to the parietal lobe of the cerebral cortex. However, information about proprioception goes to the cerebellum, which is the area of the brain responsible for motor control of the body. Signals from specific parts of the body are sent to the specific parts of the brain responsible for processing information about that area—studies that record electrical activity in the brain in response to stimulation of different body parts have shown that the brain has kind of map in it, called the *somatotopic map*. The amount of brain tissue devoted to different areas of the body is dependent on the amount of sensory input that is coming from the different areas, and this is related to the importance of those areas to a particular species.

For humans, somatosensory input from our hands is more important than somatosensory input from some other areas, such as the back, and because we have approximately one hundred touch receptors in each of our fingertips, our somatotopic map for our hands is much larger than the somatotopic map for the back. After the hands and fingertips, the most sensitive areas in humans are the lips, face, neck, tongue, and feet.

For dogs, sensory information from the face appears to be very important, and 40 percent of the canine somatotopic map is devoted to it, especially the area around the upper jaw. Other important areas are along the spine at the base of the tail. Apparently, the feet also rank high on the priority list of dogs since the somatotopic map for this area is large—dogs have many touch receptors in their pads, sensitive to vibration, which may give them information about running speed. They also have many somatosensory receptors in the webbed spaces of the feet and between the pads—anyone who has tried to spread a dog's toes for a nail trim can attest to the sensitivity of this area!

There is one type of touch receptors that dogs have but humans do not—these are specialized receptors at the base of the stiff, thick, deep-rooted hairs called *vibrissa* located on the face. They are what most people call whiskers and are more than just cute—they help dogs "feel" their way around. Since they project from the face around the eyes, muzzle, and cheeks, they are bent by the slightest contact with nearby objects, and, like a lever, the degree of bend is amplified at the deeply rooted base to stimulate tight clusters of receptors, which, in turn, trigger sensory pathways to the brain. This is a kind of a "second sight" for dogs, who, as you have learned, have poor near vision, and it alerts dogs to the presence of objects near their face, aiding in navigation in places like the burrows of prey, and for protection of the eyes from injury. Vibrissae even have their own set of muscles that direct them forward while the dog is running to provide an early warning for collisions. Vibrissae are so important to dogs that each vibrissa actually has its own somatotopic map. Cutting off the whiskers seems to impair the navigation ability of dogs, so, when you take your dog to the groomer, make sure you specify your preferences about whisker trimming since many groomers trim them to give the face a cleaner look, and disregard the functional impairment that it will cause. So, unless you want to hear your dog go "clunk" in the night, don't let her whiskers be trimmed!

The sense of touch exists to protect us—and to connect us. It gives us physical feedback about the world in which we live so that we know how to negotiate it safely. If we, and dogs, didn't have thermoreceptors, our skin would get burned or our toes would fall off from frostbite. If we didn't have chemoreceptors, which give us information about the levels of oxygen and carbon dioxide in our bodies, we wouldn't keep breathing. If we didn't have proprioception, we wouldn't know where our feet were when we tried to flee a predator—and we could trip and get eaten! And without pain, we wouldn't learn to be careful, and we would keep injuring ourselves, possibly until we died. Lack of mechanoreceptors would keep us from knowing how hard to press the accelerator in our cars, or how hard to hug people before we crush them—it would also keep us from feeling the loving touch of our mothers, our children—and our dogs.

Touch is essential to life and to love—and this appears to be as true for dogs as it is for people. At birth, puppies are blind, deaf, and have a very immature sense of smell, but, as soon as they leave their mother's body, will reliably find their way to their mother's milk supply using the thermoreceptors in their muzzles to detect the warmth of their mother's body. They nuzzle and paw the nipples to stimulate milk flow, and their mother licks them to clean them and keep them warm. This early touch forms emotional bonds between mother and puppy, and early touch between human and puppy can help form interspecies bonds that will last the lifetime of the dog. Children and puppies deprived of touch develop similar emotional and behavioral problems, including an inability to relate to others. The consequences of touch deprivation have even been found to include changes to physical health by causing damage to the immune system and gastrointestinal tract.

Recent research in humans has shown that the brain has developed two distinct pathways for processing touch information. The first, as described earlier, processes and defines the facts about touch—whether an object is hot or cold, hard or soft, round or square—and builds up a tactile image of the object.

The second pathway deals with the social and emotional information about touch and this is detected by a different set of receptors in the skin, then is processed in different areas of the brain—the ones devoted to pleasure, social bonding, and pain. The touch receptors in the skin that are specialized to detect a touch from another person—or perhaps a dog—are *C-fibers*, sometimes called "caress fibers." They connect to an area of the brain called the *posterior insula*, which is involved in perception and motor control, and we perceive the touch as a soft, pleasant sensation. Touch seems to trigger the release of endorphins, oxytocin and other hormones that cause changes in heart rate, blood pressure, muscle tone, and ultimately reduce stress while increasing the sense of emotional well-being. For humans, touch in the form of therapeutic massage is thought to relieve pain, aid in recovery from addiction, decrease depression, improve cognitive function, increase mobility, decrease anxiety, and relieve headaches, insomnia, and digestive problems.

Studies on dogs in shelters have shown decreases in heart rate, blood pressure, and stress hormones such as cortisol after the dogs have been petted by humans—even those they had never seen before. Petting dogs seems to have a two-way benefit—humans who pet dogs also exhibit lower blood pressures, heart rates, and stress hormone levels, and it is possible that those same C-fibers are responsible. Less work on that second, emotional, sensory pathway has been done on dogs—mostly due to the inability of dogs to sit still in a functional MRI machines—but there are so many similarities between humans and dogs in the first sensory pathway, as well as in the importance of touch and social bonding, that it seems likely that many parallels exist. I believe that you and your dog will find more ways to connect and communicate with each other through the sense of touch than through all four of the previously described senses of vision, hearing, smell, and taste—especially when some of those other senses begin to diminish with age. According to the surprisingly poetic Plato: *Every heart sings a song, incomplete, until another heart whispers back. Those who wish to sing always find a song. At the touch of a lover, everyone becomes a poet.* Go ahead—be a poet.

10

BLUE DOGS

There's a long life ahead of you, and it's going to be beautiful, as long as you keep loving and hugging each other. —Yoko Ono

A few years ago, just when I was thinking about writing this book, I heard a story on National Public Radio about the "Blue Zones"—these are pockets around the world where some of the most long-lived, yet healthy, people can be found.[1] In these Blue Zones, people reach age one hundred at rates ten times greater than in the United States. These longevity hotspots were identified by demographers using census data to pinpoint regions with the longest life expectancy, and, in 2004, National Geographic and the National Institute on Aging began a research partnership with writer Dan Buettner, who visited those five areas to discover whether these "super-agers" had any lifestyle characteristics in common that could explain their longer, healthier lives. At first glance, it would appear unlikely that the centenarians in Okinawa, Sardinia, Greece, Costa Rica, and Loma Linda, California, would have much in common, but Buettner found that the lifestyles of all the Blue Zone residents shared several specific characteristics, which, in his book, *The Blue Zones: Lessons for Living Longer from the People Who've Lived the Longest*, were summarized as the "Power 9" practices. These were:

1. *Moderate, regular physical activity*—No going to the gym for these people—they naturally exercised almost continuously because of the way their houses or environments were made and the work that they did.

2. *A strong sense of life purpose*—They had a clear goal in life, a reason for getting out of bed in the morning, and a sense that they made a difference by being alive.
3. *Reduced stress*—Although most of these people had lives that many Americans would not consider easy or comfortable, they took the time to slow down to enjoy and savor their lives.
4. *Moderate caloric intake*—On average, these people consumed at least 20 percent fewer calories than most Americans.
5. *Diet*—Plant-based diet, with lots of vegetables, legumes, and nuts, but limited meat and no processed foods.
6. *Limit alcohol*—Moderate alcohol intake, especially of red wine.
7. *Engagement in spirituality or religion*—They all had faith, whether it was ancestor worship in Okinawa, Catholicism in Sardinia and Costa Rica, or Seventh-Day Adventism in Loma Linda.
8. *Engagement in family life*—Those that built their lives around their family had lives filled with ritual, duty, and togetherness, and had a built-in social network that kept them mentally sharp and physically healthy—and supported whenever they weren't.
9. *Engagement in social life*—These groups of centenarians all had strong social ties with their communities—for work, relaxation, support, and the sharing of mutual interests and values.

After I heard about the ways that these groups of people lived longer and better, I wondered if some of those "Power 9" principles could apply to dogs and be a source of a greater lifespan and healthspan for them, too. Obviously, some of these nine practices are not applicable to our canine companions—red wine is definitely out, as is involvement in religion, and there are specific dietary needs of dogs that are different than those of humans—but what about the rest? The "life purpose" principle, for example—dogs were, after all, originally bred for certain purposes, and your own dog has many inborn traits that are ripe and ready to be used. Dogs that can find a way to use their instincts in a constructive way, and are then praised for it, could become more satisfied with life, knowing that they have pleased their owners, and develop a "sense of purpose," couldn't they? As an added bonus, they would also get more exercise and have less stress—two more principles down! And here's another one that applies to dogs—moderate calorie intake. Research on dogs has shown that caloric restriction has a significant effect on longevity—restricting your dog's calorie intake by 20 percent could actually lead to a 20 percent increase in his longevity!

What about engagement in social life? Well, dogs are social crea- tures—they have a sense of social structure within packs and families, and develop bonds with other dogs and people. Those that engage in activities outside their home will encounter other dogs, along with their owners, at the dog park, at doggie daycare or even just on the daily walk—and I think these dogs are more stimulated, less stressed, and probably happier than solitary dogs that never go out of their house or yard. What about engagement in family life? Most dog owners consider their dogs to be part of the family—and I think that feeling goes both ways. Families represent the most fundamental type of social network and are the type most integrated into our lives, from beginning to end. I think dogs can develop a sense of family based on how we live with them, how we treat them, how we care for them—and how we love them. They definitely build their lives around us, and we certainly give them rituals, duty, and togetherness. And what about you? Maybe your dog puts you into the Blue Zone in some ways—doesn't he provide you with a reason to get up in the morning, an incentive to exercise, a pathway to social engagement, a source of stress reduction, and a sense of family? Unless you worship at "The House of Dog," he can't help you with religious engagement, and I certainly hope he doesn't drive you to drink or stress eat, but the rest of the Power 9 principles could certainly apply to you through your very own Blue Dog. Bet you never thought that little four-legged bundle of joy you brought home a while ago could actually help you live longer!

Why is this important? Well, because aging is inevitable—it is part of the development that begins for all of us in the womb, continues through childhood/puppyhood, through the adult years, and into the years beyond that. Certain conditions are indeed more common as dogs age, and we must expect them, anticipate them, prepare for them now, and then make some compromises for them at the time needed. The key isn't to *stop* aging—the months and years will pass no matter what we do—the key is to take steps now to preserve functionality, and, later, to focus more on the abilities—and less on the chronology.

Again taking human aging as an example, I know a ninety-four-year- old man, Joshua, who still goes to work every day—he is a successful grain broker and monitors rapidly fluctuating grain prices minute by minute using five computer monitors—definitely more than I could do at my age now. Sadly, I also know a sixty-year-old woman who is in a nursing home after a disabling stroke. For these two people, their actual age in years is not as important as their ability to achieve their daily tasks in life. Sure, the ninety-four-year-old may not be able to hear as well as he used to, or get up from a chair as quickly and easily as he did when young, but he compensates for those changes with a hearing aid and some tall chairs. Although his genes and his environment also played an important role, the seeds of his successful aging were sown when he was younger because he obtained exercise, good nutrition, and good medical care, and found a fulfilling job, a strong social and family structure, as well as a variety of hobbies—so Joshua is a good example of a Blue Zone–type super-ager. My friend in the nursing home has not, of course, been in absolute control of her health destiny, since the genes she inherited were not of her choosing—but the fact that she smoked, was overweight, and had high blood pressure prior to her stroke were important contributing, and, probably, controllable factors.

How does this relate to your dog? Well, health is both a nature and nurture phenomenon. You can't control the nature part—your dog's genetic hand was already dealt long before you were on the scene. However, you, the owner, are the one with the type of brain that allows you to educate yourself about your dog, choose the right food types in the right amounts, learn how to control his environment, provide him with preventative health care, and give him a social structure, a sense of family, as well as a goal in life. This means you have the power to provide the majority of the nurture part of this equation. Joshua did that for himself. He keeps himself involved in his work, his family life, his social life—that way, he keeps himself active physically and mentally. Dogs don't have the cognitive abilities to do this for themselves—and that is where *you* (and I) come in. So, instead of the "Power 9," I have devised some Blue Dog principles, designed to help you help your dog live longer and live better, that I call (with apologies to the Beatles) the "Fab 4":

1. provide purpose
2. supply structure
3. target togetherness
4. practice prevention

11

PROVIDE PURPOSE

If you don't mind throwing tennis balls for eternity, I do have an opening in doggie heaven. (Angel at St. Peter's Gate, to a man seeking admittance) —*Frank and Ernest* comic strip

Give your dog a job. I'm not kidding. And never let retirement happen. Remember Joshua from the previous chapter? He didn't, and his mind and his body have benefited from that. Using the information presented earlier, think about what your dog's breed (or, if you have a mixed breed, what you guess your dog's breeds to be) was created for, and combine that with what you now know about your dog's personality. Choose activities that would appeal to those inborn instincts and could fit with his personality, then tap into that innate desire to perform those functions. Start these in puppyhood, and keep doing them throughout your dog's life. This will give you and your dog something to do together that will be enjoyable, provide exercise for both of you, provide mental stimulation for your dog, and open up a social structure for you both to depend on throughout life. Habits and routines are good to develop while your dog is young, since your dog, when he is older, will continue to anticipate them *and* will want to participate in them for many years. You, and these activities, will give your dog a reason to get out of bed in the morning, so his body and his brain will never turn to mush.

Now, I realize that not all people can sign up their Australian Shepherds for sheep-herding sessions with a local flock of sheep or go hunting with their retrievers, but, first, you'd be surprised how many local groups are offering these sorts of things on the weekends, and, second, if you are unable to participate in those activities, how easily you can do something similar—like throwing the tennis ball or hiding it for a game of hide-and-seek—which can approximate certain activities if you are informed and creative, and aware of your dog's abilities, personality, and instincts.

If you are interested in organized sports activities for your dog, there are an astonishing number of dog sports in which you and your dog can participate. The list of sports these days is dizzyingly long, in fact—from the traditional (obedience training and conformation showing) to the esoteric ("dogrobatics" and "muskrat racing")! Trust me, many sports that you never dreamed existed will probably be available somewhere near you—just read through some of the sports and their descriptions in this chapter, and conduct an online search—you'll be amazed! Most of these sports involve some basic obedience training but otherwise just simply appeal to the prey drive of all dogs, while, at the same time, use their acute senses of hearing and smell.

Certain sports tap into certain talents that are strong in certain breeds, such as tracking, retrieving, or running, and the key is to figure out what your dog's special talents and abilities are and then match him (and you) with a sport that you would both enjoy. Think about the original purpose for your dog's breed or breeds, and how certain activities might not only appeal to your dog, but fulfill him. Think about what you now know about your dog's personality—some dogs are suited for team sports, and some are not. There is no shame in this—some people are happier when they engage in competitive team sports, while others enjoy more solitary sports when they only compete against themselves to achieve their personal best. It's all about what fits, and what brings out the best in your dog—just remember that not all dogs conform to their breeds' stereotypical talents, since humans have been breeding for appearance more than ability in recent years. "Think outside the breed" when considering what might fit your own dog.

Do you have a dog that likes water? Try "Dock jumping"! Do you have a dog that likes to dig or tunnel? Try "Earthdog"! Is your dog a dedicated squirrel-hunter? Try "Barn Hunt"! See if you can match some of these sports to your own dog's interests and talents:

- *Agility*—a handler directs a dog through an obstacle course in a race for both time and accuracy.

- *Barn Hunt*—for this there is a simple maze of straw bales, with plastic tubes hidden in the maze containing live rats. The dog must climb on a bale with all four feet, go through a tunnel, and alert the owner to the rat, by barking or sitting down—and the fastest one to do that wins. (Don't worry—the rats are family pets of the participants and are experienced at this game, knowing they are safe inside their little ventilated tubes.)
- *Canicross/Caniteering*—a cross-country running competition with leashed dogs.
- *Competition obedience*—a dog sport in which a dogmust perfectly execute a predefined set of tasks when directed to do so by his handler.
- *Conformation showing*—individual purebred dogs are judged by how well they conform to the established breed type for their breed.
- *Disc Dog*—the competitors in this sport are judged by the height and speed at which the dog can catch a flying disc thrown by the handler.
- *Dock jumping*—this one is simple: dogs jump into the water, and they are judged on how well they do. Variations of Dock jumping exist, too:

  - *Big Air*—the dogs' jumps are measured for distance.
  - *Extreme Vertical*—the competitors jump to snatch a dog toy suspended eight feet over the pool.
  - *Speed Retrieve*—the dog is judged by how fast she swims when fetching a thrown object.
  - *Iron Dog*—the holder of this title has won the combination of all three!

- *Dog Parkour* (also called Urban agility)—the competitors perform the agility-type activities of climbing, jumping and balancing using obstacles typically found in an urban environment.
- *Earthdog trials*—these involve man-made underground tunnels that the dogs must navigate, while scenting a quarry, such as a rat.
- *Field trials*—a competitive event at which hunting dogs compete against one another; there are separate field trials for retrievers, pointing dogs and flushing dogs.

- *Flyball*—teams of dogs race against each other from a start/finish line, over a line of hurdles, to a box that releases a tennis ball to be caught when the dog presses the spring-loaded pad, then back to their handlers while carrying the ball.
- *Herding or stock dog*—competitive dog sport in whichherding dogs move sheep around a field, fences, gates, or enclosures as directed by their handlers.
- *High jumping*—just like the sport for humans, the dog is judged by the highest hurdle he can clear.
- *Lure coursing*—involves chasing a mechanically operated lure, usually a plastic bag, across a field.
- *Mushing*—this is a general term for any sport that involves a transport method (such as a sled, cart, bike, or skis) powered by dogs and includes Carting, Pulka, Scootering, Sled Dog Racing, Bikejoring, Skijoring, Freighting, Wheelchair Mushing, Urban Mushing and Weight Pulling.
- *Musical canine freestyle*—a mixture of obedience training, tricks, and dance that allows for creative interaction between dogs and their owners.
- *Nosework*—a canine sport created to mimic professional detection tasks.
- *Obedience trials*—the participating dogs are judged by their compliance with the commands given by the handler.
- *Protection sports*—these are obedience and protection sports which include Schutzhund, French Ring Sport, American Ring Sport, and Mondio Ring Sport.
- *Racing*—in this sport, the need for speed is what counts; there are breed-specific racing events for Dachsunds, Terriers, Greyhounds, Whippets, and Sled Dogs.
- *Rally obedience*—the dog and handler proceed at their own pace through a course of designated stations; each of these stations has a sign providing instructions regarding a skill that is to be demonstrated.
- *Retrieving trials*—these simulate hunting conditions where the dogs' ability to retrieve is tested over various terrains and conditions using artificial game.

- *Sheepdog trials (or herding)*—this is a competitive dog sport in which herding dogs move sheep around a field, fences, gates, or enclosures as directed by their handlers.
- *Surfing*—yes, surfing—there really are competitions for dogs that are trained to surf!
- *Tracking trials*—this competition uses the dog's ability to use the sense of smell to locate a lost person or article.
- *Treibball*—a herding competition (without sheep) in which the dog must gather and drive large exercise balls into a soccer goal.
- *Water Sports*—these are sports that demonstrate skills at a variety of tasks in the water, including "Nautical Nosework," "Aquagility," retrieving, diving, towing, and water rescue.

Having your dog engage in activities that he knows he is good at, and that *he* knows *you* think he is good at, can actually improve your relationship in unexpected ways. I saw a client, Barbara, recently with her little mixed-breed rescue dog, Murphy, that she had adopted a year ago. When I first examined Murphy just after he was adopted, I could barely touch him—he cowered at the sight of me and would then lunge to bite me without warning. This did not bode well for our relationship, despite the fact that he was my namesake! However, when I saw him recently, I did the whole exam, complete with vaccines and a blood draw, without incident. I was astonished at the transformation and asked Barbara how this miracle had occurred—she told me that she had been taking him to agility classes, and that the experience of training Murphy for this sport had caused them to bond in a way that she had not experienced with her other dogs. She said that, since Murphy needed to look at her for direction and leadership during training, he had started to look at her for direction at other times. The positive reinforcement he got during training, especially when he did well, gave him confidence and this had generalized to times outside the agility setting since he realized he could get positive reinforcement for good social behavior elsewhere. In addition, the exercise relieved his stress while the sport had given him an outlet for his nervous energy. Knowing how he was last year, I wouldn't have thought agility would have been a good fit for his personality or his body, especially since Murphy doesn't look like a dog one might associate with dog sports or athleticism. He is an adorable little shaggy guy with huge ears, whose DNA analysis revealed to be 50 percent Pomeranian, 25 percent Poodle, and 25 percent unidentifiable mixture of several breeds. But it would have been better if I had kept an open mind—agility both fit him and benefitted him.

As you consider activities for your dog, in addition to taking your dog's personality and instinctual talents into account, you also need to be aware of any breed-related physical risk factors that could lead to injury, illness, or long-term damage to your dog's body. Those dogs with hip dysplasia, for example, are at risk for arthritis if they repeatedly jump in the air to catch a flying disc and land on a hard surface. Each landing on hips that don't fit tightly together will cause a little movement within the joints and will beat up the cartilage lining the joints— over time, this repetitive concussive trauma leads to arthritis. Brachycephalic dogs—the flatter-faced ones like Bulldogs, Boxers, and Pugs— have a hard time keeping their bodies cool, and will overheat more easily during activity than other breeds of dogs. These dogs are not good candidates for activities that require sustained running or even walking without frequent opportunities to rest, drink, and cool down. This does not mean they can't be active—it just means they require owners that have knowledge about their abilities as well as their limitations and wise choices can then be made to keep them both stimulated and safe.

Much of the information on dog breeds, dog sports, and local activities is available in a variety of books, on specific breed-fancier's websites and websites devoted to certain sports. However, keep in mind that several other activities exist for the nonsports-minded, or the nonsports-abled, that can provide you and your dog with a mutual interest, a shared sense of purpose, and many social interactions. Think about visiting nursing homes, hospitals, shelters, or hospices—many of my patients and clients do this, and all parties seem to benefit greatly. Small breeds of dogs, such as Shih Tzus, Cavalier King Charles Spaniels, and French Bulldogs were originally intended to be companion dogs—even though they were descended from ancestors that performed other tasks, such as protection or hunting, these scaled-down versions were intended to provide comfort and love. The calm, loving demeanors of many large dogs make them good candidates for the role of therapy dogs—remember the Golden Retrievers that were present to help the surviving schoolchildren in Newtown, Connecticut, in 2012?

The natural canine instinct to bond and support humans is a benefit all dog owners can reap—why not spread a little of that love around?

Different facilities have different requirements, but all require some basic obedience training as well as screening by the program coordinators regarding the temperament of the dog and reactivity to things like IV poles, wheelchairs, or walkers. Some facilities require certification by programs such as Canine Good Citizen (akc.org/dogowner/training/canine_good_citizen/links.cfm) or the Delta Society (deltasociety.org). Passing the series of tests required for these certification programs requires some specific training, and many dog training centers throughout the country have classes geared toward these tests.

Another way to provide your dog with a sense of purpose, some exercise and lots of mental stimulation right in the comfort of your own home is to do a little Lumosity-style brain training—and you can do a little citizen science at the same time. There is an amazing website called Dognition (dognition.com) which was developed by Dr. Brian Hare (author of the book I mentioned earlier, *The Genius of Dogs*) along with many other researchers in the field of canine cognition. "Cognition" is the activity of thinking, understanding, learning, and remembering. This website contains interactive games that you can do with your dog that give you information about how he understands the world, while allowing you to understand him. These games are not meant to test your dog's intelligence, but to discover what his individual gifts are, and for you to use them to keep him mentally and physically stimulated—so you can both have fun! An added bonus of this is that all the results of hundreds of these tests are aggregated and used for research on canine cognition and behavior (the first paper using the data generated by these citizen scientists was published in September 2015).[1]

When you subscribe to dognition.com (which is a fee-based service), the first thing you'll do is complete a Dognition Assessment, which is a group of twenty games (don't worry, they walk you through them with instructions and videos), and then you receive your dog's Profile Report, which gives you information about your dog's thinking style and individual talents. Then, each month you receive a new game to complete with your dog, setting the way to have new things to do and new things to learn. I think this is a great tool for you to use, and who knows—you and your dog might just advance our human understanding of that species with which we are so familiar, but of which we are so very ignorant.

12

SUPPLY STRUCTURE

The chains of habit are too strong to be felt until they are too strong to be broken. —Samuel Johnson

What if you don't have time for organized sports and activities? You can develop habits. Everyone develops habits. Some can be healthy (routinely brushing our teeth twice a day, for example), some can be annoying (my lack of neatness), and some can be pathologic (obsessive-compulsive conditions). But, in general, most of us rely on habits to structure our days and make life predictable and safe—and so do dogs. That predictability can be very comforting over the years to dogs as they get older. Your dog very quickly learns your personal routine—such as when you get up or go to bed—and learns to join in with it. Your dog will also learn when you leave for work, when you will return home, when walks are scheduled, and when mealtime is. These events will be anticipated with either excitement or anxiety—and you may anticipate them with the same enthusiasm—unless of course, your dog annoys you by waking you up early every morning in anticipation of breakfast! Taking your dog for a walk every day, twice a day, doing a short play session, a short obedience routine every day, a little daily grooming, and a little tooth-brushing are not only healthy activities for you and your dog, but also can give your dog something to rely on when the senses of hearing, smell, and vision diminish with age.

One of the best habits you can develop is to simply teach your dog tricks and do them every day. This requires little time, no money, and no travelling. Years ago, I thought that making dogs perform tricks was silly, was somehow degrading for the dogs, and just a way for the humans to show their superiority. Then I moved to Washington, D.C., and was fortunate enough to live near the National Zoo. During one of my visits there, I saw someone running the seals through a series of tricks, rewarding the successful performance of each with a delicious chunk of stinky raw fish. This shocked me and I was somewhat indignant about it—after all, this was the *National Zoo*, not a circus! Catching sight of one of the trainers, I strode up and asked why these seals were being forced to do these demeaning tricks—and what he said has come to mind so many times since then: he said that the seals that ran through a routine series of tricks every day were less bored, got more exercise, displayed less aggression, were more cooperative with each other, and seemed to look forward to their training sessions. I realized that the tricks were not so insulting to the seals after all, but gave *them* a reason to get up every day and promoted positive social engagement (maybe they were Blue Zone seals). Whether or not you already participate in lots of activities outside your home, develop a repertoire of tricks for your dog and do them twice a day at least. It is fun, amusing, develops a bond between the two of you, helps increase your cooperation as a team, and provides at least a little exercise.

My parents did this with their dog—none of the three of them were inclined to do much walking, but my parents faithfully ran their Cavalier King Charles Spaniel, Tory, through her ten basic tricks every evening, and followed that with three throws of her ball (not two, never four). Tory lived to be a perky fourteen-year-old and saw my parents into their mid-eighties. My parents went through a fairly basic list of tricks with Tory but it never failed to delight all three of them every single night! The actual repertoire of "tricks" doesn't really matter, as long as there is an established repertoire and routine. Your dog will look forward to this daily interchange of commands, praise, and rewards, along with the accompanying sense of mutual satisfaction. You may want to come up with a checklist of tricks that are appropriate to your dog's interests, skills, and activity level, as well as yours. It's the routine, the habit, the *job* that you and your dog need—this is a part of the scaffolding that will support and structure your lives together for the next decade or so. Tory never got too old to do this job, and she never retired from her profession of delighting my parents—I really do think she knew she had a purpose because of these practices. These habits and routines can be restructured as time goes on to accommodate for changes in your dog's mobility and motivation, but, ultimately, their value is to provide your dog with the social interactions that studies in human senior citizens show to be beneficial for a long, mentally active life.

These habits and activities will be helpful for your own Blue Zone aspirations as well, since routines will give you and your dog exercise, a job, a strong sense of family ritual and social structure, and some stress relief. I have noticed over the years that dogs who are nervous when they come into our clinic will calm down if their owners have them perform their little repertoire of reliable tricks. Once the dogs focus less on the unfamiliar environment and more on this familiar ritual, you can see them relax and can feel their confidence growing as they perform, knowing that they will receive not only a treat, but great praise and applause. There are several books available that describe at-home games and tricks to teach your dog—two that I can recommend are: *101 Dog Tricks: Step by Step Activities to Engage, Challenge, and Bond with Your Dog* by Kyra Sundance and Chalcy, and *Play with Your Dog* by Pat Miller. In both, the tricks are fun, the instructions are clear, and all training is, as it should always be, based on positive reinforcement.

When my dog, Jersey, lost some of her hearing as she grew older, she gradually started doing things that she would never have done before—like snatching food off a table, or grabbing an expensive shoe and running off with it. The more I thought about it, the more I was convinced that she had started to "misbehave" for two reasons: first, she could no longer hear anyone in the house and she thought she was alone when she got food off the table or grabbed my shoe; and, second, she could no longer hear the word "No!" and she had free rein to do anything she wanted! The flip side of hearing loss for Jersey, I also realized, was that she also never heard me say "Good girl!" anymore, or any of the chatty things I always said to her as I did things around the house. I realized then that the loss of hearing for a dog, who does not have the ability to understand that it is a normal part of aging, would be very isolating. I was regretful at that time that I had not thought ahead when Jersey was a puppy and taught her the hand signals for "Good girl!" and "I love you!" (as well as "No!" and "Drop It!" of course!)—but I have certainly done so with Jersey's successors ever since.

When you start training your new puppy, and while you are perform-ing your daily routines with your adult dog, remember that your dog will not always have acute hearing as aging occurs. Teaching hand sig-nals for certain basic commands will be easy while your dog is able to hear, but pretty difficult after hearing loss has already occurred. It doesn't really matter what the words or the gestures are—but they do need to be consistent and clear. All you need to do to teach hand signals to pair with those commands is to perform specific, very easy-to-see (as your dog's vision may become somewhat less acute with age as well), and very distinct gestures at the same time that you are teaching your dog the verbal commands.

Perform the hand signals before you say the commands, and always, always, always follow the dog's successful performance of the desired behavior with a food treat—behavioral studies in dogs show that dogs learn more quickly with the use of food treat rewards along with praise, than with praise alone. Dogs, as a species, have a very strong food drive (they wouldn't survive long in the wild without it), and you can take full advantage of that throughout your own dog's life. Make the food re-wards for training especially desirable for your dog—after all, most of us would perform somersaults for great chocolate, but maybe not try so hard for a celery stick—and make those rewards small and frequent. And, in this case, size truly doesn't matter!

First, some general guidelines about the teaching of hand signals: pair a verbal command with a hand signal, giving the hand signal just before the verbal command, and, when your dog performs the desired action, immediately give him a treat. Dogs readily make associations between things—but timing and repetition are the keys. Dogs live in the here and now, and if you wait too long between the command, the action, and the reward, an association may be made with something totally unrelated that just happened to occur at the time of the reward, such as the backfiring of a car or a knock on the door!

After you have repeated and promptly rewarded the correct action several times, you can start eliminating the verbal command, while sometimes using the verbal command alone and sometimes using the hand signal alone, rewarding your dog each and every time it is done correctly. Once your dog reliably performs the correct action in re-sponse to either the verbal command or the hand signal, you may also gradually eliminate the food reward, although I think it is best to use treats often, in order to continue to solidify the association as well as the good (and fun!) consequences of performing this repertoire in the years to come.

Remember to be consistent about which hand is used for each signal and maintain stable use of body language, eye contact, as well as "tone" of command, whether it be tone of voice (loudness, firmness, happiness) or tone of hand signal (the gesture's clarity, emphasis, enthusiasm).

And, now, here is a short list of commands and hand signals that you will find useful for the years to come—having these signals securely in your dog's repertoire while hearing is still acute may save you some annoyance, if not grief, in the future. By the way, these signals might come in "handy" in situations where there is lots of background noise, or when you don't want to make any noise at all, like when someone is sleeping.

1. *Sit*—Start with your dog standing in front of you. Hold a treat on or in your fingers (with your palm up) and, starting with your hand at your side, bring it up, folding your arm as if you were going to toss the treat over the same shoulder. Do this slowly, bringing the treat past your dog's nose. Say "sit" at the same time. You're leading his nose upward as you say sit, and the body's weight will naturally shift toward the back end so sitting often occurs automatically. When it does, enthusiastically praise and give the treat. Repeat, and repeat, and repeat. . . . You will, eventually, be able to signal-command your dog to sit with just the gesture of raising your hand from side to shoulder with the palm up and fingers straight, without the verbal command and without the treat.

2. *Down*—Start with your dog sitting in front of you. Hold a treat in your fingers and, with your hand raised above your head, bring it down, keeping your arm straight until it is hanging at your side. Do this slowly, bringing the treat past your dog's nose as you signal. Say "down" at the same time thus leading the nose down while you say the command. When your dog lies down, praise and give the treat. Repeat, repeat, and repeat . . . and the gesture will eventually become the command.

3. *Come*—Start with your dog in front of you. Hold a treat in your fingers. Start with your arm held straight out to your side parallel with the ground. Now sweep your arm forward so your hand touches your opposite shoulder (as if you were throwing salt over your shoulder for luck!). Do this slowly at first, bringing the treat past your dog's nose as you signal. Say "come" and back up a few steps at the same time. When your dog comes toward you, praise and give the treat. Repeat—well, you get the idea.

4. *Good Dog*—This one is the easiest to teach, but also one of the most important to have in your repertoire for later on when your dog can't hear your praise! Start by choosing any sign you'd like to use, such as "thumbs up." Then teach it by sitting with your dog while holding a handful or so of really tasty treats. Use your "Good" sign, and give the dog a treat. That's it—except for the repetition part! Once you give your "Good Dog" sign and your dog looks at you as if to say: "Hey, where's my treat?" you're solid!

5. *Watch Me*—Teaching a command for, and rewarding your dog for, eye contact is one of those investments of time that pays off now as well as later. Now is a good time to get your dog in the habit of looking at you for direction, so your dog will still pay attention to you during distractions. Later, due to decreasing hearing, it might otherwise be difficult to get your dog's attention for the hand signals and commands, unless your dog has already developed the habit of watching you. Start by taking a treat, put it up to your dog's nose, bring it up to *your* nose, sign and then say: "Good dog!" and then give the treat. The idea is for your dog to look you in the eye. Practice this for a few days. Then hold the treat away from you (start out a foot or so from your face). Your dog will probably look at the treat. Wait until your dog gets impatient, and looks at you to say "well, where's my treat?" Quickly sign "Good Dog!" and give the treat. At first, all you will get is a quick glance, but you can slowly build up the time that your dog will look you in the eye. You should also hold the treat in different places (use the other hand, hold it in front of you, and at full arm's length, even behind your back). You want your dog to learn that no matter where the treat is, the only way to get it is to look at *you*.

6. *Free Dog*—Teaching a release command is very important, especially if you plan, as I recommend, to teach the "stay" command
   later. If you do not tell your dog that it's OK to move or do
   something else, your dog will make the decision, not you. It is a
   fairly simple instruction to teach. Whenever you finish practicing
   one command, sign "Free Dog" before going on to the next. Do
   this by making a circle with your forefinger and thumb, extending
   the remaining fingers upward like the "OK" sign. When you end
   a training session, always sign "Free Dog," and then put away the
   treats.

7. *Stay*—Have your dog sit and sign "stay" using your hand held
   with the palm in front of the dog's face. Quickly give a treat, then
   sign "stay" again, another treat, "stay," and one more treat. Then
   say and sign an enthusiastic "Free Dog!" and you are both done—
   for now—since you both need to change positions. Gradually
   make the time between the treats a bit longer, so your dog will
   stay sitting for longer periods of time (still use three treats, and
   then a "Free Dog!" when done working). Once your dog seems to
   understand, move on to the next step. Gradually add some distance (keeping the treats near you, pick each one up and bring it
   to the dog). Do not try distance and duration at the same time. If
   you want your dog to remain in the "stay" position longer, you
   should stay nearby. If you want to increase the distance between
   you, keep the duration of the "stay" short. Be sure to use your
   release sign, so that your dog knows when to move. Once this
   command, the sign, and the desired response are well established, add in some distractions during the "stay" period, like
   having another person come into the training area or tossing
   around some tempting toys.

8. *Stop It*—Since "No" is a very overused word in dog training, what
   you really want to teach with this hand signal is "Stop It *Now!*"
   This should only be used for very serious infractions of good
   behavior, since you want your dog to *really* pay attention to you at
   the time needed. This is a command that you will have to teach
   when something happens spontaneously that you do not like, and
   you should accompany the gesture with a firm verbal command
   of "Stop It!" along with body language and a facial expression that
   indicates your deep displeasure. *Do not* physically punish your

dog. The best, in my opinion, gesture to use for this command is something like the "Safe" signal that baseball umpires use—for this, they start by crossing their arms at the wrists, and then quickly uncross them in a very broad, dramatic motion.

9. *Drop It*—Teach this command and signal to get your dog to let you take an object from his mouth. This is a very important safety command for the (hopefully) few times that something dangerous is taken, like a chicken bone or a bar of chocolate. Gather a few of the safe objects that you know your dog likes to chew on. Have a piece of food ready in your free hand, held in your fingers with your palm up, as you tempt your dog to chew on one of the desirable items held in the other hand. Once the item is taken, put the treat very close to your dog's nose and firmly say, "Drop it." Give praise when the object is relinquished. Feed the treat as you pick up the item again with your other hand. Return the item to your dog. Repeat (of course!) through several repetitions and with several different objects. However, after the verbal command is well engrained, occasionally "pretend" to offer the treat once the test object is dropped, using the now-empty fingers of your free hand, with the palm up. Do this without the treat more and more often and—presto: the hand signal for the command "Drop It!" (your empty fingers with your hand palm up) will have already been learned!

10. *I Love You*—This, of course, is my favorite. After all, as the song says: "The greatest thing you'll ever learn, Is just to love and be loved in return." You and your dog learned *that* a long time ago, but this way you can learn how to continue to show it and, there-fore, for him to continue to know it, over all the years to come. This signal is one of the American Sign Language (ASL) signs, and is done with the hand raised, palm forward, and the third and fourth fingers curled against the palm. This one will be *very* pleasurable for you to teach and for your dog to learn! Just give this hand signal just before saying "I love you!" and then do whatever you want to show it—this is the one signal that will not need a treat to reinforce it! That will happen by the very nature of your relationship. How easy is that?

Above all, these training periods should be pleasant, fun, fairly short, and extremely rewarding for both of you. Don't work for so long that either of you gets bored or frustrated, and do give rewards early and often. All dogs really care about, and what most dog owners care about, is the act of giving and receiving something that makes their loved ones happy. Repetition of this simple exchange many, many times during each and every day, whether during sports, tricks, or just the reinforcement of your own unique shared habits, will give you and your Blue Dog the social structure, family ritual, and mutual support that might help age-proof the both of you. And guess what? *This* helps satisfy Blue Dog Fab 4 principle no. 3: "Target Togetherness"! Just remember, it's all about the relationship, always and forever.

13

PRACTICE PREVENTION

Youth is the gift of nature, but age is a work of art. —Stanislaw Lec

When we start a journey, we have a much better chance of arriving at our destination if we have an itinerary and a map—or at least Siri! Avoiding wrong turns, traffic jams, and construction zones makes the trip not only more pleasant, but also safer. As you contemplate your dog's path through life, it helps to know how he'll get through it, what kinds of health problems he might encounter, and what health pitfalls to avoid.

Back when I was a physician assistant in the field of pediatrics, I performed routine well-child exams in addition to exams for medical problems. After performing a physical examination on the child, I also asked the parents certain questions to uncover health problems or developmental delays that might not be apparent in the strange, scary environment of the exam room. Your veterinarian will be relying on you for this kind of information about your dog. Your regular home physical exams, your attentiveness to any changes in his personality and behavior, and your ongoing awareness of the status of his five senses will allow you, and your vet, to have early warning of potential health problems before they actually *become* problems.

There was one other aspect of routine well-child checks that I was taught, and I have always thought that it should be part of veterinary well-dog exams—this was an assessment of safety hazards for each child. Was the child in the right type of car seat? Did the parents smoke? Is there lead paint in the home? Was there a pool that the child could fall into? Did the parents use sunscreen on the child? Was there a gun in the house, and where was it kept? These were routine screening questions, not meant to be invasive, but to find out things that could be the difference for that child between life and death, between healthy lungs and asthma, between a healthy brain and a damaged one. During routine veterinary care visits, veterinarians, like pediatricians, should also perform safety checks for dogs—after all, many of the same health risks exist.

Did you know, for example, that smoking around your dog can raise his risk of nasal and throat cancer as well as chronic lung inflammation and even skin allergies? How about sun protection? Dogs with white fur, especially those that have very short fur, can get sunburned on their ears, noses and backs—this raises the risk of skin cancer, just like it does with humans. The best thing to do is prevent prolonged sun exposure, but you can actually use sunscreen on your dog, as long as it doesn't contain zinc, which can be toxic to him. What about pools and ponds on or near your property? Every year, dogs drown after falling in pools while unsupervised—unless their owners have taught them ahead of time where the steps are to climb out of the pool.

Did you know that allowing your dog to ride in the front passenger seat could kill him? If you have an accident, and the airbags deploy, they will save your life, but could crush your unrestrained dog as he flies forward and the bag inflates toward him. If he is in the back seat, but unrestrained, during an accident, he could become a projectile that can crash into you, into the windshield, against the back of your seat—even out the window! It is much safer for your dog to be restrained in some manner in the car. There are a few ways to do this. One is to have him ride in a dog crate, as long as the crate itself is tethered tightly and securely to the car's floor or backseat. In the event of an accident, he will still hit the side of the crate, but his chances of injury are lower because of the shorter distance. If you don't want to use a cage, there are several brands of padded safety harnesses to purchase—these attach to the seat belt, and most dogs will accept them if they are introduced in short sessions with lots of positive reinforcement. For the little dogs, car seats are available—these are really little padded platforms that have a harness incorporated in them. The little ones seem to like them—they allow a better view—but the seats still need to be installed in the backseat if the car has a passenger seat airbag.

Now, one more very important tip—in order to be as proactive as possible about your dog's health, it is crucial to be aware of any risk factors that he has for certain health problems—now or later in life. A risk assessment is a process by which you identify hazards, analyze, or evaluate the risk associated with that hazard, and determine appropriate ways to eliminate or control the hazard. Performing a risk assessment on your dog allows you to be proactive about his potential health hazards, so you can eliminate or control their long-term consequences. It pays, after all, to take the long view on your dog's health, since what you do now can change the trajectory of your dog's pathway to old age, and can determine what kind of life he—and you—will have at that time.

Most risk factors for the health of humans as well as dogs involve a combination of genetic predisposition and environmental influences. Diseases such as cancer, diabetes, heart disease, and asthma have been found, in humans, to "run" in families—individuals in those families may be born with certain genetic mutations, or certain combinations of genes, that set the stage for certain diseases later on. Some individuals will go on to develop those diseases and some will not—and that is because their genes can be modified—turned on or off—by exposure to certain chemicals in their environments, or by lifestyle choices such as smoking, drinking, or obesity. Similarly, many canine diseases are genetically based and "run" in certain breeds, or even in certain families within breeds. It is estimated that up to 40 percent of purebred dogs have genetic defects that will likely affect their health at some time in their lives.

As your dog's caretaker and health-care advocate, you should become familiar with the genetically linked problems he might have inherited. If you educate yourself about the problems to which your dog's breed is predisposed, you'll know what to watch for in your own dog, how to avoid problems when possible, which diagnostic tests should be employed during routine wellness visits, and which treatments are available for any conditions that might develop. For example, Wheaten Terriers are prone to a kidney problem called *protein-losing glomerulo-nephropathy* that leads to chronic protein loss in the urine, and can lead to kidney failure. If you own a Wheaton and know that he is prone to this disorder, you can ask your veterinarian to perform a urine test every year that detects how much protein is in your dog's urine, allowing you to catch this disease in the early stages when it is most treatable using diet and medications.

As another example, Labrador Retrievers are genetically predisposed to hip dysplasia—if you know about this breed-related predisposition, you can ask your vet to take hip X-rays while your Lab is a puppy or young adult to identify any signs of poorly formed hips before any problems have developed. Hip dysplasia is a disease in which the ball and socket components of the hip joint are malformed—the ball portion and its socket don't properly meet each other, resulting in a ball that wiggles more within the socket, and that rubs and grinds instead of sliding smoothly. Over time, this chronic extra motion and grinding leads to new bone formation—also known as arthritis. The degree of the arthritis that develops is dependent, in part, on the weight carried on the hips—the higher the body weight, the more concussion those unstable joints undergo, and the greater the arthritis that develops. If you know, early on, that your dog has hips prone to arthritis, you might be more serious about weight control throughout your dog's life, and you could tailor your dog's activities and lifestyle to prevent the consequences of this genetic predisposition. Corrective surgery could even be done if the hip dysplasia is severe—but most of those procedures can only be done when a dog is young. If the dysplasia is less severe, being careful to avoid activities that jolt the hips (such as jumping up to catch a ball) and using supplements to nourish the hip's joint fluid (glucosamines and dietary fatty acids, such as fish oils) will lessen the degree of arthritis your dog experiences. This may not seem as important now, as you gaze at your healthy-appearing, bouncy young puppy—but will be essential when your dog reaches the teen years, since the ability or inability to walk can be a life-limiting factor for older, large-breed dogs.

By the way, you don't even need to know the breed of your dog to assess some health-risk factors—certain disorders are dependent on body shape, or conformation. An example of this is the tendency for certain dogs to develop a disorder called *gastric dilatation volvulus* (GDV), commonly known as "bloat"—this is a very serious condition that occurs when the stomach becomes distended with air and then twists around on itself. This interferes with the blood supply to the stomach and other digestive organs, and blocks the passage of food, leading to worsening bloating. The distended stomach slows down the return of blood to the heart, decreasing the amount of blood the heart can pump and decreasing the blood pressure. Without blood to supply oxygen, tissues start to die, releasing toxins into the blood stream which cause serious disturbances in heart rhythms—a common cause of death in these dogs. Dogs most susceptible to GDV are the large breeds that have deep, narrow chests, in which the stomach appears to be more mobile within the abdomen. Other factors that increase the risk for GDV include overeating, rapid eating, single daily feeding, high water consumption, stress, and exercise after eating. Examples of genetically predisposed breeds include Great Danes and Irish Wolfhounds, but I have seen this in breeds as diverse as Golden Retrievers, Standard Poodles, and Basset Hounds.

This condition is a true emergency with, unfortunately, a low survival rate after a great deal of pain—but is actually easily preventable by a surgical technique called *gastropexy*. In this, the side of the stomach is tacked, using sutures, to the side of the abdomen, and prevents enough movement of the stomach to keep it from turning over on itself. Most veterinarians in general practice can perform this surgery at the time of a dog's spay or neuter surgery—in our practice, it is done laparoscopically so that the incision is smaller, but this technique requires special training and special equipment that is not available in every veterinary clinic. Those owners of susceptible dogs that have the right information about their dog's health risks can do so much to, at least, minimize the consequences of them, and, at most, save their dogs' lives—this example of GDV and its preventative surgery is a classic illustration of my favorite motto "Forewarned is forearmed"—but you can't be forearmed if you aren't forewarned.

Go ahead, forewarn and forearm yourself early on in the life of your dog by identifying his genetic predispositions to certain diseases. What are the health hazards related to his breed or body shape? What are the risk factors that might allow those hazards to become health problems? Write them down, along with any symptoms to watch for, any tests your veterinarian could do that could help identify them or monitor them, and then think of ways that *you* can be the environmental influence that *won't* allow that genetic predisposition to be expressed. Then, during your monthly health evaluations on your dog, perform a brief risk assessment, too, and then evaluate how well you are, or are not, helping him avoid or control his individual health hazards.

For example, if you know your Lab has hip dysplasia, how are you doing with his weight control? Have you remembered to give his joint supplements? If you have a Wheaton Terrier, are you noticing any changes in his water consumption or urine output that could indicate kidney problems? Is he losing weight or is his muscle mass decreasing, which are also signs of kidney disease? If you have a Great Dane, are you feeding three to four small meals with rest afterward or two large meals with exercise afterward?

All of this may sound daunting, but this information is available from your veterinarian as well as on several reliable websites. The website I would suggest checking out is the Canine Inherited Diseases Database, compiled by the Atlantic Veterinary College, University of Prince Edward Island, and the Canadian Veterinary Medical Association at ic.upei.ca/cidd. To use the database, type in the name of your dog's breed, or the name of a disorder, in the search box at the top of that webpage. Each breed page lists the more serious and common disorders in that breed that are thought to have an inherited component, and each disorder is linked to the appropriate disease page. On each disorder page, you will find a description of the condition, information about how the disorder is inherited, consequences of the condition for you and your dog, and the recommended care by you and your veterinarian. By being proactive about your dog's health risks early in life, the road to his later years will be so much safer and more pleasant for both of you.

Unfortunately, some health problems—breed-related or otherwise—will happen anyway, and your veterinarian will help your dog get through them. But who will help *you*—and your wallet—get through them? That's when having health insurance for your dog comes in handy. There are many good plans, with varying premiums and coverage, and you can find more information about the different ones on the website petinsurancereview.com/dog. I highly recommend signing your dog up for insurance, especially before any "preexisting conditions" are found—having the means to pay for treatment of an emergency illness can mean the difference between life and death for many dogs. Assessing your own ability to pay for the treatment of certain health problems in your dog is, therefore, another way of doing a health risk assessment on your dog. Take that one seriously—and look into health insurance.

Along with the health hazards your own dog has as an individual, there are potholes in the road of life that all dogs, of all breeds, will encounter and it will be beneficial for you to learn about them as well, in order to help your dog dodge them, too. Two of these are presented next.

UNIVERSAL HEALTH HAZARD NO. I: OBESITY

There is truth to the saying that "Rich, fatty foods are like destiny: they too, shape our ends." OK, so maybe you were expecting something a little more exciting than a discussion about weight control. But remember, we are trying to increase not only the longevity of your dog, but also your dog's ability to enjoy and utilize all those extra years. Weight control is a *huge* topic—so to speak—in the news, in human healthcare, in politics, for insurance companies, and in our everyday lives. Recently, I searched on the Internet for the term: "obesity epidemic"—and pulled up 1,700,000 results! Obesity is defined as an abnormal accumulation of body fat, usually 20 percent or more over an individual's ideal body weight. The Center for Disease Control (CDC) released these statistics for the United States in 2014:

- Percentage of adults age twenty years and over who are obese: 34.9 percent
- Percentage of adults age twenty years and over who are overweight (and not obese): 34.4 percent

For dogs, obesity is the most common nutritional disorder in the United States, and is estimated to include 25–40 percent of the dogs in this country. In one recent study, an overweight owner was three times more likely to have an overweight dog. It is easy to see that, as the percentage of overweight Americans increases, which is predicted to occur (estimated to be 42 percent of Americans by 2050), as will the percentage of overweight American dogs. How could this be? After all, dogs don't get seduced by fast food commercials, order pizza, and drink giant cups of corn-syrup-laden soda! Humans, the ones with the smarts, control their diets completely and would *never* make our dogs into "obeasts"! Well, there is a problem with that assumption—most dog owners do not perceive their dogs as obese, and many veterinarians fail to acknowledge obesity as a disease and don't discuss it—especially if the dog owner is obese. In addition, many dog owners are not aware of the health risks related to obesity—well, all that is about to change for you.

Fat: What Is It Good For?

Well, *not* "absolutely nothin'"! Fat accumulates for good reasons—it helps humans, dogs, and other species store excess calories in a safe way so that those calories can be mobilized for use during times when calories are not being consumed. In addition, fat releases hormones that control metabolism. Fat is now, in medical circles, being referred to as an "organ"—which is defined as a somewhat independent body part that performs a special function. Despite our dislike of our fat, it is an entity worthy of "big" respect!

Fat: What Is It Made Of?

There are four types of fat—brown, white, subcutaneous, visceral, and belly fat. Brown fat is now thought to be more like muscle than like white fat. When activated, brown fat burns white fat. In recent studies in humans, scientists have found that lean people tend to have more brown fat than overweight or obese people. Children have more brown fat than adults, and it helps them keep warm. Brown fat quantities decline in adults but still help with warmth. The job of white fat is to store energy and produce hormones that are then secreted into the bloodstream. Subcutaneous fat is found directly under the skin all over the body, including the limbs, trunk, and abdomen. Visceral or "deep" fat wraps around the inner organs. And then there is "belly fat"—this seems to be the one that is always popping up online in those annoying, belly-jiggling animated online ads I never asked to see—and there seem to be endless diets, supplements, and cures for it. Belly fat is actually comprised of both visceral and subcutaneous fat, which means that, luckily, there is not a fifth type of fat to worry about. Apparently, one gains weight first within the visceral/abdominal area, and then the subcutaneous fat around the abdomen increases. This is important, because that means the abdominal/visceral fat is the last to go when weight is lost.

Fat: What Is It Bad For?

A lot! Here are a few disorders in dogs that are definitively linked to excess body fat and excess weight:

- earlier age of death (not exactly a disorder, but kind of disabling)
- pressure on the windpipe (tracheal collapse)
- pressure on the diaphragm (expiratory airway dysfunction)
- reduced oxygen supply to the heart (myocardial hypoxia)

Here are the many disorders for which overweight or obese dogs are predisposed:

- lower urinary tract disease due to bladder stones
- cardiovascular disease
- kidney disease
- oral disease
- cancer—breast and bladder
- blood clots in the liver (portal vein thrombosis)
- hip dysplasia
- arthritis
- ligament tears in the knee (ACL rupture)
- shoulder damage (humeral condylar fractures)
- "slipped" discs in the back (intervertebral disc disease)
- high blood pressure (hypertension)
- reduced immune function
- inflammation of the pancreas (pancreatitis)
- insulin resistance
- constipation
- incontinence (in female spayed dogs)
- skin problems
- increased risk of complications from anesthesia and surgery
- reproductive problems
- high blood fat levels (hyperlipidemia)

If you go to the National Institute of Health's website (nih.gov) and search for the health risks for humans related to obesity, you will find a shockingly similar list—obesity in people leads to an increased risk of conditions such as cardiovascular disease, high blood pressure, arthritis,

diabetes, dementia, and some cancers, as well as, unfortunately, prema-
ture death. Some of these problems are related to the production of
chemical and hormones by the biologically active fat, and some are due
to the presence of the fat causing mechanical changes in the body. For
example, visceral fat releases the hormone *leptin*, which plays a role in
appetite regulation but also in learning and memory. Researchers spec-
ulate that, in excess, leptin may have some adverse effect on the brain
and could be the reason that obese humans have a greater risk of dementia.

The physical space taken up by fat can cause health problems, too.
For example, although dogs don't get the atherosclerosis (hardening of
the arteries) and resultant heart attacks that humans have in association
with obesity, dogs get heart problems because of the presence of excess
fat around the heart, which restricts its movement, and, therefore, function. Dogs can also develop breathing problems related to excess weight
in the abdomen, as this "belly fat" restricts the movement of the diaphragm, which is the muscular wall below the ribcage that contracts
and expands the chest cavity, and, thus, the lungs. This is known, by the
way, as Pickwickian syndrome, named after a character in Charles Dick-
ens's *The Pickwick Papers*, who was a fat little boy who ate large quantities of food and fell asleep all the time. In humans, and probably dogs,
this condition leads to lower oxygen and higher carbon dioxide levels in
the blood, causing chronic sleepiness.

Overweight dogs have a high incidence of arthritis, since the degree
of arthritis that joints develop over time is directly impacted by the
amount of concussive trauma they get over time. The greater the
weight, the harder the impact on the joints every time their feet hit the
ground and the greater the wear and tear on the cartilage within the
joints over time. Do this experiment—weigh yourself, multiply that
weight by 0.20, then take a backpack, fill it with some household items
that add up to whatever that weight was, and then put the backpack
on—you are now obese! Carry this extra weight around for a few hours,
running up and down stairs, doing household chores, getting up from a
chair. See how tired your back gets, and how sore your feet and ankles
become over time, how out of breath you get as you go upstairs—and
don't let your dog experience this kind of mechanical trauma over his
lifetime!

There's a pretty easy fix for this. Pay attention to how many calories your dog gets every day. It's not rocket science—just addition and subtraction, although I suppose rocket scientists do that. First, find out how many calories your dog's current food contains per cup—it is usually listed on the website for the food manufacturer or, sometimes, on the bag. Then, try to figure out all the sources of all the nonmeal calories your dog receives in a day. This includes rawhides, dental treats, table scraps, treats for going outside—*everything*. You don't need to stop giving him all those things—after all, giving those treats and watching him enjoy them is an essential part of your relationship—you just need to be aware of what they are, so you can modify them (not eliminate them) if need be.

If your dog, based on your physical exam that you are doing regularly, is getting heavier according to changes in his body condition score, reduce his calories by 10–20 percent, in part, by trimming a few calories from those treats. Use Cheerios, for example, instead of dog biscuits—at 120 calories per cup, they are less caloric—and dogs think they are getting something really special!

Also, reduce the calories fed in the meals by reducing the amount of food you are giving by 10–20 percent or, better yet, find a food that contains 10–20 percent fewer calories per cup and feed the same amount. However, it is often nutritionally better to find a food that is intended for weight loss than it is to just reduce the amount of a "regular" food. The weight loss foods are nutritionally balanced despite the decrease in calories, and reducing the amount of "regular" food to eliminate calories might also eliminate nutrients for your dog. Look for a food that is at or under three hundred calories per cup—dog foods can be anywhere from 250 to 550 calories per cup! Be aware that the name and flavor of the food will have very little to do with how many calories it contains. I've seen "weight control" diets that are more caloric than "maintenance" diets, and fish-based diets that are more caloric than beef-based ones. Every time you change flavors or brands, you will be changing the number of calories you give your dog, so always check the label or the website for the food before you do so.

By the way, once your dog is an adult, do *not* pay attention to the feeding guidelines on the bag—they are almost always too high. If your dog is not losing weight despite using a lower-calorie food, you'll have to reduce the amount you feed. Pieces of dry dog food are like little calorie bombs—each one is extremely calorie dense—after all, the water has been extracted to make the food convenient for us humans to store and feed, and this concentrates the calories into a very small space. You can easily give your dog extra calories without even knowing it by using a "rounded" cup of food instead of a level one. If you are using a cup measure (and you should be), take Taylor Swift's advice and "Shake it off!"—that is, shake it a little from side to side after scooping and a few kibbles will fall off if it isn't level. This may not seem like much, but a rounded or heaping cup of food could contain one-eighth to one-fourth cup extra food—feed this twice daily every day for a year, and that's 12.5–25 percent more calories, and, potentially, 12.5–25 percent extra weight!

I read somewhere that, if we adult humans consume one hundred extra calories per day for a year, we will gain ten pounds! One hundred calories sounds like nothing—especially when you stare at one of those one-hundred-calorie cookie packs while you are in the grocery line, but one hundred calories is significant. A moderately active woman between the ages of thirty-one and fifty should consume about two thousand calories per day—one hundred calories is 5 percent of that. Add that number of extra calories over a long time—which is how most gain weight without knowing it—and the weight goes up correspondingly.

The good news is that eliminating that number of calories over time can allow you to lose weight, too, without severe diets or feeling deprived. The same is true for dogs. Reduce in lots of small ways, and it will add up—or is it subtract down? Your dog won't take well to sudden, severe caloric restrictions—that is a recipe for lots of counter surfing and begging at the dinner table, but he won't notice many little, subtle reductions over time—like giving him a third of a dog biscuit instead of a whole one when he comes in from outside. After all, your dog can count—he knows he'll get a treat every time—but he can't do fractions!

Other ways to reduce the number of calories going into your dog include changing *your* perceptions about how much, or how little, you are feeding your dog. When I feed my twelve-pound terrier her one-fourth cup allotment of food, it looks like a lot more to me when I put it in her little tiny bowl than when I put it in my Golden Retriever's huge bowl—I might feel a little sorry for her every time I feed her if it looks like too little food, and I might inadvertently give her a couple of extra kibbles to make up for her deprivation. Studies in humans show that we will eat more if our food is on a large plate than on a smaller one—this probably happens when we feed our dogs, too. If you're feeling a little sorry for your dog every time you feed him his paltry cup of dry kibble, you probably are adding a little extra food without realizing it.

Try this—the "Five Kibbles Out Diet"! Feed your dog whatever you usually feed him—and then take back five to ten kibbles, depending on the size of the meal. Those kibbles each represent a large portion of the total number of calories in that bowl—one cup of my dog's average size kibble contains two hundred kibbles (yes, I counted them)—removing ten removes 5 percent of the kibbles and 5 percent of the calories. Somehow, it's easier than feeding less in the first place—if you're like me, you won't be able to stand measuring out less than a cup, but it doesn't seem so bad to just take a few back off the top of the bowl. Over time, this little maneuver will make a difference!

There is, of course, another part to the equation—we've talked about how calories go into your dog (courtesy of you, actually) but how do they go "out"? Well, they get used for energy to drive all the cells in our body at all times as long as we are alive—when we move, breathe, sleep, even think. This is our metabolism, which is the way our body transforms energy, as supplied by calories. A *calorie* is actually a measurement of units of heat energy, and is defined as: "the energy needed to raise the temperature of 1 gram of water through 1°C." Many people use the term *kilocalorie* interchangeably with calorie. The difference is that a kilocalorie is the amount of energy needed to raise the temperature of a larger amount of water—one kilogram—by one degree Celsius and is equal to one thousand calories and is the unit most often used to measure the energy value of foods (I will only use the term "calorie").

One's metabolic rate is the rate at which our bodies burn calories to get the energy needed to maintain vital functions like breathing, pumping our hearts, circulating our blood, maintaining a normal body temperature, keeping our brains alive, and our internal organs functioning. Part of what determines each individual's metabolic rate is the muscle mass or lean body mass. Other factors include age, gender, the amount of muscle in the body versus the amount of fat, the amount of physical activity, and genetic background. Some of these factors are under your control, and some are not. Your dog's genetic traits are fixed, but you can have an influence on the degree and manner of their expression, as we've discussed before. Your dog's gender is not under your control, but you do need to be aware that reproductive status—that is, whether your dog is spayed or neutered—has a big influence on the metabolic rate. Dogs that have had their testicles or ovaries removed, which removed most of the sex hormones, testosterone or estrogen, will have a 35 percent decrease in their metabolic rate. That's big—and not being aware of that can make your dog big, too! Once your dog is a young adult, you need to take this into account when choosing foods for your dog.

The other major factor that influences metabolic rate, physical activity, is totally under your control, as is the proportion of fat to muscle in your dog's body. This is why giving your dog a job, with the physical activity that accompanies it, is so important. In humans, exercise is more likely to be done if it is fun or if there is a social aspect to it—that helps dogs, or at least their own human personal trainers!

UNIVERSAL HEALTH HAZARD NO. 2: DENTAL DISEASE

I know, I know—it's not that exciting. But bear with me—it is incredibly important—taking care of your dog's teeth now and throughout life has profound consequences in parts of the body that are distant from the mouth. You will, of course, want your dog to have teeth for as long as they are needed for eating, chewing on toys, and smiling at you—but you will also want your dog to have healthy kidneys, a healthy heart, and a healthy brain for as long as possible. In dogs, there is a link between dental disease, kidney function, and heart disease, and, in humans, dental disease has also been shown to be associated with conditions that affect the kidneys and heart, as well as others that affect the brain, liver, lungs, skin, and joints. How does this happen? First, it is helpful to understand what we are talking about—and below are some definitions.

Periodontal Disease

Periodontal diseases are actually a group of chronic inflammatory diseases that affect the tissues that support and anchor the teeth. Left untreated, periodontal disease results in the destruction of the gums, alveolar bone (the part of the jaws in which the teeth are imbedded), and the outer layer of the tooth root. The tissues that are involved are the *gums*, which include more structures than we usually think: the *gingiva*, the *periodontal ligament*, the *cementum*, and the *alveolar bone*. The *gingiva* is a pink-colored mucus membrane that covers parts of the teeth and the alveolar bone. The *periodontal ligament* is the main part of the gums. The *cementum* is a calcified structure that covers the lower parts of the teeth. The *alveolar bone* is a set of ridges on the jaw bones (the maxilla and the mandible) in which the teeth are embedded. The main area involved in periodontal disease is the *gingival sulcus*, a pocket between the teeth and the gums.

Gingivitis

Gingivitis is an inflammation of the outermost soft tissue of the gums in which the gingivae become red and inflamed, lose their normal shape, and bleed easily. Gingivitis may remain a chronic disease for years without affecting other periodontal tissues. Chronic gingivitis may lead to a deepening of the gingival sulcus, which can then allow the teeth to become loose.

Periodontitis

Periodontitis is the most serious form of the periodontal diseases. It involves the gingiva, the periodontal ligament, *and* the alveolar bone. A deep pocket forms between the teeth, the cementum, and the gums. Plaque, tartar, and debris from food and other sources collect in this pocket. Without treatment, the periodontal ligament can be destroyed and destruction of the alveolar bone can occur. This allows the teeth to move more freely and they can eventually fall out. The mechanisms by which bacteria in the periodontal pocket cause tissue destruction in the surrounding region are not fully understood, but several bacterial products that diffuse through tissue are thought to play a role in disease formation. Bacterial endotoxin is a toxin produced by some bacteria that can kill cells. Studies show that the amount of endotoxin present correlates with the severity of periodontal disease. Other bacterial products include proteolytic enzymes, which are chemicals that digest the protein found within cells, thereby causing destruction of those cells. The immune response has also been implicated in tissue destruction. As part of the normal immune response, white blood cells enter regions of inflammation to destroy bacteria. In the process of destroying bacteria, periodontal tissue is also destroyed.

Gingivitis usually results from inadequate oral hygiene. The bacteria responsible for causing gingivitis reside in plaque—plaque is a sticky film that is largely made from bacteria. Tartar is plaque that has hardened—and plaque can turn into tartar in as little as three days if not brushed off. Tartar is difficult to remove by brushing. The key is to brush your dog's teeth while the bacteria-laden plaque is still soft enough to be brushed off—that is, at least every three days. Twice a week—that's not so hard, is it?

Now let's talk about how much of the teeth you need to brush. Not how many of the teeth—you need to brush as many as possible—but how *much* of the tooth surfaces. The teeth in dogs are shaped differently than those of humans—dog teeth are more crescent-shaped than human teeth, which are blockier. This means that there is proportionately more tooth surface on the outside (cheek side) and inside (tongue side) of the teeth, and less surface area in between teeth as well as less

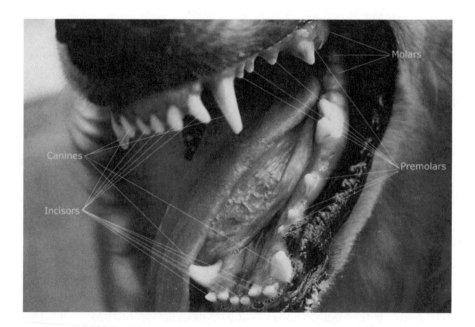

Figure 13.1.   The Four Major Groups of Dog Teeth. Thinkstockphotos.com/*phviola*.

contact between the teeth. That is why humans need to floss between teeth, as the brush bristles can't get in there, and one reason why we get cavities, which dogs do not. I am sure you will be happy to know you do not need to floss your dog's teeth, and you will be even happier to know that you only need to brush the *outer* surface of your dog's teeth—since the flat inner surface of dog teeth is kept clean by the dog's tongue! Isn't this getting easier and easier?

As shown in figure 13.1, there are four main groups of teeth to brush: the *incisor* teeth (the small teeth in the very front), the *canine* (fang) teeth, the *premolar* teeth (along the sides), and the *molar* teeth (far in back). It is important to brush all four areas, although it may be difficult to see the last (the fourth) premolar and the two molars way behind the corner of the mouth. You don't really need to see those teeth to brush them—just remember they are back there and reach way back under your dog's cheek to reach them.

And what do you use? Definitely do *not* use human toothpaste— some contain a sweetener called Xylitol, which, if ingested by a dog, can lead to low-blood sugar (hypoglycemia). Also, all human toothpastes contain fluoride, which, because it will be swallowed by your dog (if someone out there trains a dog to swish and spit, please let me know), can, over time, cause changes in the blood levels of calcium and magnesium, irritation of the stomach and intestines, changes in heart rhythm, lethargy, and lack of appetite. Most of us, and our dogs, are already getting some fluoride from our water supply and the products we consume that contain fluoridated water. Any additional fluoride can be a problem for our dogs. The other reason not to use human toothpaste is that most dogs hate it! All the things that are put in toothpastes to get humans to enjoy using them—such as the mint flavoring (mint is in the bitter category, and, as you know, dogs hate bitter) or the foaming agents—backfire when it comes to dogs. Luckily, many more palatable (to dogs, anyway) products are available. Most are flavored to dogs' liking—such as chicken, beef, peanut butter, or malt. Brushing will be a rewarding experience for one and all! There is even bacon-flavored toothpaste for dogs—one of my clients told me that her kids swiped it from their dog's little medicine cabinet thinking bacon-flavored toothpaste sounded like the best idea ever! Luckily, she found where it was hidden in the bathroom before they used it. Many pet toothpastes also contain enzymes that help break down that nasty, sticky plaque on the teeth before it turns into tartar. Some are slightly abrasive and will help, along with the friction of the brush, take off tartar that has already formed. Many brands of pet toothpastes are available at your veterinarian's clinic, pet stores, or online pet suppliers.

By the way, there are many, many dental products available for dogs—but they are not regulated in any way, and may not live up to their labelled claims of effectiveness. There is one organization that tests dental products and awards a "seal of acceptance" if the products meet their claims. This is the Veterinary Oral Health Council (vohc.org) and you can go to its website for lists of effective veterinary dental products.

Now that you know a bit about toothpaste, you need to know about brushes—you can use a human toothbrush (as long as you don't get it mixed up with your own!), but, since human toothbrushes are angled in such a way that we *can* brush all the surfaces (i.e., bent forward), you may find it easier to use a toothbrush specifically designed for dogs. These brushes are bent backward, as you will be standing facing your dog, and your arm and hand will be at a different angle than they are when you are brushing your own teeth. Some dog toothbrushes have a small head, some have a large head, and some have one of each at either end! There are also "finger toothbrushes," which are rubbery, thick caps with bristles on one side that fit over the tip of your finger—some dogs will accept their owner's finger in their mouths (especially if they have been trained to do so as puppies) more than a funny-looking plastic stick with bristles! I have a friend who uses two finger toothbrushes for what she calls "The Double-Scrub Blitzkrieg"—she puts one brush on each forefinger, puts a little toothpaste on both and then, standing facing her dog, puts one finger on each side of her dogs mouth all the way to the back of the back teeth, and brushes simultaneously from the back to the front. She does this so fast that the dog never seems to have the time or the inclination to react! Whatever method, brush, or toothpaste works for you and your dog is the one to choose—as long as the job gets done!

I bet you're wondering how long you need to brush your dog's teeth. Humans are supposed to brush all reachable tooth surfaces for two minutes, twice daily, every day. You, on behalf of your dog's teeth, only need to worry about plaque removal on the outer surfaces of the teeth, and that only takes about ten seconds. Let's do a little math here:

humans, ideally, are supposed to brush all surfaces of our teeth for two minutes twice daily, seven days a week, and floss twice daily. Dog owners need to brush the outer surface of our dog's teeth for about ten seconds twice weekly. I have just cut your work down by an amazing amount—1,680 seconds per week just brushing our own teeth versus twenty seconds a week brushing our dog's teeth! Does that sound all that difficult, really?

Start early in your dog's life—with brief sessions at first, stopping *before* your dog starts to struggle or gets overwhelmed. Simply put your finger alongside the teeth on the side and slide all the way back until your finger can't go any further (most people don't realize how far back in the mouth some of those teeth are), praise your dog, pop in a treat, and go on with your day. Fairly quickly, your dog will sit still a little longer each time, and have positive associations with this new activity. Then, try using a little toothpaste on your finger to let him taste it, then give him a treat without making a fuss. Next, try the finger toothbrush with a little paste, for just long enough for him to feel the texture of the brush, then pop in the treat—well, you get the idea. Remember to give your dog the positive reinforcement *before* you get to the point where there is any negative response from your dog, since once there is a struggle, you have already lost the opportunity to provide a positive experience for the mundane, yet very important, activity.

So why, again, should you be doing this? Well, you would want to prevent tooth loss, for obvious reasons, and, of course, you want to prevent any discomfort your dog could get because of chronic gum inflammation, periodontitis, and loose teeth. Also, for your own sake, you probably wouldn't want to smell your dog's bad breath while you're spending quality time together—those teeth become nasty-smelling due to all that bacteria growing on and around them! But even more importantly, those mere ten to twenty seconds twice a week are an investment in your dog's long-term future health and longevity.

Since you now know something about the anatomy and physiology of periodontal disease, it will be easier for you to see how dental disease can have an impact on organs in the rest of the body. Fewer studies have been done in dogs than in humans, so less conclusive evidence is available. In humans, however, associations have been detected between periodontal disease and hardening of the arteries (atherosclerosis), heart attacks, complications during pregnancy, diabetes mellitus, blood vessel abnormalities, and increased levels of C-reactive proteins, which are proteins carried in the bloodstream that are released during inflammation (some physicians measure this protein to assess a patient's risk of a heart attack). Studies done on dogs after death revealed that dogs with moderate to severe periodontal disease had changes in the heart muscle (myocardium), heart valves, the kidneys, and the liver, compared to dogs with less severe periodontal disease. In both humans and dogs, bacteria are released into the bloodstream to circulate around the body (this is called bacteremia) whenever there is disruption of the surface of the gums, which includes processes such as benign as chewing and tooth brushing. If there are lots of bacteria on and under the gum tissue, and if the gums are themselves inflamed and fragile, it follows that more bacteria are released from unhealthy gum tissues than healthy gum tissues.

It is suspected that frequent transient bacteremia, combined with chronic stimulation of the immune system, plays a role in the development of systemic disease. A study done in 2011 measured C-reactive protein levels before and after dental cleaning and found that the levels of C-reactive proteins correlated with the severity of periodontal disease, and that these levels decreased after the teeth were cleaned.[1] It is important to note, however, although many associations have been found between periodontal disease and pathologic organ changes in dogs, no studies have been done yet that show exactly how one causes the other.

Some of the bacteria and debris from the infected mouth tissue can enter the blood stream. Blood circulates everywhere, and certain areas have been found to "trap" that debris and bacteria. A study was done in 2008 in an effort to correlate the extent of periodontal disease with the likelihood of damage to organs such as the kidneys, liver, and heart. The amount of periodontal disease "burden" was estimated by the depth of the periodontal pocket (the one that can form between the teeth, the cementum, and the gums). For each centimeter of periodontal disease burden, there was a 1.2–1.4 times greater likelihood of damage to the valves within the heart, as well as to the liver and the kidneys.[2]

Brushing your dog's teeth is one of the most important, simplest, and most logical components of good dental care for your dog, but it requires a multimodal approach—similar to good dental care for humans. Getting plaque *off* your dog's teeth while the plaque is still soft is the best way to prevent the accumulation of the tartar that the plaque will eventually become—but what else can be done to prevent the plaque from bonding to the tooth surface in the first place? Well, there are water additives that can be mixed with your dog's drinking water that can do that! Several dry "dental" dog foods have been developed to do this—these are generally made to crumble less when chewed, since food crumbs can stick to plaque, accumulate on the tooth surface, and provide a tasty meal for both your dog *and* the bacteria in your dog's plaque! Check the Veterinary Oral Health Council's website to see which foods have been evaluated, and, of course, consult your veterinarian as well.

What about chew treats? This is a low-maintenance way to help keep your dog's teeth clean—for this, you can take advantage of two things: your dog's innate, species-driven desire to chew, and the fact that the majority of the teeth in your dog's mouth were originally meant to shear meat off of bones. But you also have to take advantage of your wisdom, as a human, to choose the right things for you dogs to chew on. Dogs will chew on almost anything (as you and your furniture may have already discovered) but they don't always chew—or choose—wisely. The Goldilocks principle of dog chew treats is as follows: some chew treats are too hard, some are too soft, and some are *just right*.

Too Hard: Bones, Antlers, Hooves, and Inflexible Nylon Bones

These chew treats will indeed take tartar off of teeth, but can also take *teeth* off teeth. The teeth that are most often broken are the large teeth in the back, as these strong teeth, that have multiple roots, are what the dogs use for gnawing. Sometimes, those fractured teeth are merely chipped superficially on the tips—but they often will have what is called a "slab fracture," which is a vertical break that encompasses the outer (the side toward the cheek) portion of the tooth, and usually extends up under the gumline, and exposes the inner core (pulp) of the tooth (where the nerve is) to the bacteria in the mouth. The bacteria can then go along that channel up into the roots, which are very long in dogs, and cause an infection or even abscess way up in the cheek area, under the eye.

Too Soft: Rawhides and Pig Ears

These treats are enjoyable for your dog, and may take some plaque off of the teeth, but, while they are being chewed, they become soft and gooey. This same property that makes them digestible if swallowed, and, therefore, safer for your dog and your dog's teeth, also makes them less effective in removing hard tartar. When buying rawhides, buy ones that seem almost ridiculously, cartoonishly big—this will keep your dog busy gnawing on them without being able to tear off a large chunk and then swallow it.

Just Right: Edible Treats

The type of chew treat that is "just right" to remove tartar is the kind that is about as hard as tartar but not harder than teeth, so that, as your dog gnaws at it with those big, strong back teeth, the tartar will be scraped off. And, since your dog will chew little bits off the treat and then swallow them, this type of treat needs to be digestible. Several of these types of edible treats have been tested by the Veterinary Oral Health Council and appear on their website. At the time of this writing, the effective products include: Greenies, Check-Ups and Milk-Bone Brushing Chews for Dogs, all of which are widely available at pet stores and veterinary clinics. These edible treats come in different sizes, and the size of the treat you buy is dependent on the weight of your dog. Please watch your dog as the treats are consumed—if your dog breaks the treat in half and then swallows it whole, the treat will not help reduce tartar, as they are meant to be gnawed, and that large chunk of treat will be harder for your dog to digest. Ten seconds of brushing every other day, alternating with one edible treat every other day, will add up to fewer dental cleanings, and more years of good health, good fun, and good breath.

14

CH-CH-CH-CHANGES . . . TRENDS TO WATCH FOR IN MIDDLE AGE AND BEYOND

You may not control all the events that happen to you, but you can decide not to be reduced by them. —Maya Angelou

What is aging? Is it the gray hair and wrinkles that defines it, or is it the wisdom that accompanies it? Is it a state of body or a state of mind? Is it the clock or the cells? In scientific terms, aging is a natural, inevitable process, which begins when a life begins, and progresses through defined stages of development, maturation, and senescence. In popular terms, it seems that aging is only talked about once the *senescent* stage has been reached—that's the stage when cells stop dividing and begin to deteriorate, and the body has a harder time maintaining *homeostasis*. That term is from two Greek words—*homeo-*, meaning "similar" and *-stasis*, meaning "stable," and is defined as "the tendency of a system to maintain internal stability due to the coordinated response of its parts to any stimulus that would tend to disturb its normal condition."

As we, and our dogs, age, we gradually lose the ability to repair ourselves when exposed to internal and external stresses. This gradually leads to loss of function in various body systems, leaving us less able to fend off disease, and, eventually, leads to death. In viewing aging as a continuum comprised of these inevitable phases, it is important to realize that none of us, no matter what we do or what supplements we take, can avoid that final end point—either for ourselves or for our dogs. But we have certain choices we can make that can influence the length of those two latter phases of senescence—ideally, we want to maximize the length of time spent in the healthy aging phase, and minimize the time spent in the unhealthy, debilitated aging phase that occurs toward the end. If we can slow the rate of aging, by influencing the underlying biological processes that drive aging, we may reduce the frequency and delay the onset of many age-related disorders, or at least decrease the degree of debility they impose. This is what I mean when I invited you to "age-proof" your dog. Your dog will age no matter what you and I do—but you can, with knowledge and understanding, influence her *pattern* of aging.

What causes aging? Well, that question probably won't be answered until all of us have gone through a whole lot more of it! There are many, many hypotheses and scientists have been formulating them for more than two thousand years. One of the ways to answer that question involves asking a second one: why do different species have such vastly different lifespans? Aristotle had a theory about that—he thought that it had to do with the water content of the body. Larger creatures, like elephants, have a lot of moisture in their bodies and should take a long time to dry out and die, whereas mice would have smaller bodies, lower water content, a shorter drying time, and, consequently, shorter lifespans. This theory fell out of favor a very long time ago, but Aristotle did make an observation that remains a foundation of aging research—larger animals, at least in the wild, tend to live longer than smaller ones.

This generalization does not extend to our pets, in fact, it's upsidedown—cats usually live longer than dogs, and smaller dogs tend to live longer than bigger dogs. One branch of aging research is focused on this phenomenon, in part because our pets serve as a good model for our own aging, since they are subject to many of the same environmental influences that we are—and since we veterinarians keep more medical records on dogs and cats than on any other species. Other branches of research on the biology of aging are focused on species as diverse as yeast, fruit flies, roundworms, jellyfish-like creatures called *Hydra*, mice, naked mole rats, clams, turtles, and Zebrafish. Despite the many years of research, the mechanisms that determine aging rates among and within species are still unknown. No antiaging elixir has been found either, but some things that influence the longevity of cells have been discovered:

- *Body size*—Two theories exist about this correlation:

  - *Metabolic rate*—Smaller animals tend to have faster calorie use, faster heart rates, faster cellular turnover, and so on, than larger ones—although this one is controversial since the methods used to measure metabolic rate vary.
  - *Selection pressure*—Smaller animals have higher rates of predation in the wild, so they need to age quickly in order to reach sexual maturity and reproduce before they are eaten.

- *Dietary restriction*—Many, many studies have shown that caloric restriction, a reduction in nutrient availability that stops short of malnutrition, extends lifespan in many organisms, including dogs. Most studies have shown that a restriction of 30–50 percent typically increases lifespan by 30–50 percent. In addition to the extended lifespan, the rodents and monkeys studied have reduced rates of most age-associated cancers, do not have problems with glucose and insulin metabolism, and avoid many age-related declines in heart and brain function.
- *Telomere length*—Remember these from chapter 3? They are the protective caps on the ends of chromosomes, which get shorter every time a cell divides, and the enzyme that repairs and lengthens damaged telomeres is called *telemorase*. Telomeres were initially viewed as a kind of aging clock—the shorter the telomere, the greater the biological age, for example—but this has not proved reliable, as different people of the same age can have telomeres of different lengths. Plus, telomeres apparently influence cancer susceptibility—longer telomeres are associated with a greater risk of some cancers, and this, of course, could shorten lifespan.
- *Mitochondrial dysfunction*—Mitochondria are the so-called powerhouses of each cell, and their function is to produce energy for the cell so it can perform its own function. This theory is related to the previously mentioned theory as to why smaller animals live faster and die earlier than larger ones, and has failed, in itself, to prove a relationship between energy expenditure and life span. However, mitochondria do more than produce energy—they produce waste products of energy metabolism called *reactive oxygen*

species (ROS)—which release substances you may have heard about—*free radicals*. One theory involving mitochondria is that aging is a result of the accumulation of the harmful reactive oxygen species within the cell, which can damage the DNA within the mitochondria themselves. Another theory is that, when the mitochondria age and start to malfunction, this causes dysfunction of the cells in which they are found, with subsequent damage to the body, and aging. Although it is clear from various studies that mitochondrial function declines with age, it is also clear that this cumulative damage is not, in itself, enough to actually cause aging.

- *Stem cell health*—These are unspecialized cells that give rise to specialized cells. Stem cells within organs participate in tissue maintenance and repair after injury; research in the role of stem cells in aging is focused on three areas:

  - *Genetic mutations* in the stem cells themselves—these give rise to altered descendants of those cells, and lead to multiple accumulated changes in the cells they maintain, that then result in aging.
  - *Epigenetic changes*—These are DNA alterations which are due to the addition or removal of chemical tags called methyl groups; these can change gene expression and exert a "ripple effect" throughout the lifetime of a stem cell by giving it the wrong instructions, thus leading to aging because tissue repairs are not being made properly.
  - *Environmental factors* (that is, the environment inside the body but outside the stem cells) that affect stem cell function—This refers to the factors circulating in the body to keep the stem cells themselves healthy. If these change, the stem cells themselves age and fail to maintain and repair tissues, leading to aging. One of the interesting findings of research in this area is that, if plasma (a blood component) from young mice is injected into old mice, the stem cells in the brains of the old mice return to a more youthful stage!

- *mTOR pathway*—The mTOR protein is a *kinase* (which is an enzyme that transfers phosphate groups from one molecule to another and is crucial to cell metabolism) and it has been found that inhibition of one of the forms of this enzyme by use of a drug called *rapamycin*, originally developed as an antirejection drug for organ transplants in humans, significantly extends the lifespan of yeast, worms, flies, and mice, even if started late in life. In mice, it extends life by 13 percent in females and 9 percent in males, and has also been shown to reverse cardiac decline and improve immune function. How, exactly, rapamycin works is being actively researched—and part of this research involves its use in dogs! As part of the Dog Aging Project at the University of Washington in Seattle (dogagingproject.com), a trial is underway to assess the ability of rapamycin to promote healthy aging and increase the lifespan of middle-aged dogs. The next phase of this study will enroll healthy, middle-aged dogs in different areas of the United States who will take a low dose of rapamycin over several years, and will be evaluated over that time on the strength of their immunity, their incidence of cancer, their heart function, and cognitive abilities. Check out their website for further information on the project and to monitor the progress of the trial.

- NAD^+—This stands for *Nicotinamide Adenine Dinucleotide*, the biologically active coenzyme form of Vitamin B_3 (*Niacinamide*). During energy production, NAD^+ and NADH transfer their electrons back and forth, and thus initiate and facilitate many different metabolic processes by carrying electrons from one reaction to another. These coenzymes are needed to turn sugars, fats, and proteins into fuel for our cells. Aging research on this coenzyme centers around the changes in cellular concentration of NAD^+ that occur in aging, and attempts to change aging by changing NAD^+ use or production. One of the body's uses of NAD^+ is as a cofactor (that is, electron donor or acceptor) for other enzymes. Some of these enzymes, called the *sirtuins*, have been found to be important themselves in the deceleration of the aging process. This has turned attention to the things that activate the sirtuins— one of these sirtuin activators may actually be familiar to you—it is *resveratrol*, a component of the skin of grapes, blueberries, raspberries, and mulberries. Resveratrol is thought to be the reason why consuming modest amounts of red wine has positive health effects for humans.

- *Intestinal bacteria*—The *microbiota* of the gut is the ensemble of microorganisms which are being examined for their impact on age-related changes in immunity, muscle mass, and brain health. Studies have shown that the intestinal bacteria composition of older individuals is different than younger ones, but which aspects of this phenomenon are the cause of aging and which are the result of aging is the focus of much research at this time.

None of these aging theories alone explains the phenomenon of aging—but all of them together might do so. Aging is undoubtedly a multifaceted process influenced by multiple internal and external factors yet to be determined. This summary of research into the biology of aging was brief and very, very simplified, but I think it is helpful to be aware of it. We have a great deal more to learn about how much, or how little, we can change the aging process, and this information may be useful for you in the future to help understand new information on aging as it becomes available, as well as to help sort through some of the information—and misinformation—on the Internet about antiaging supplements.

Understanding a little about the interior mechanics of aging gives us the basis for understanding aging's external signs in our dogs. For me, when I look at my canine patients, I need to tell the difference between normal aging changes and disease states, between changes that impact the *quality* of my patients' lives and the changes that might impact the *quantity* of my patients' lives, between the things that I can alter and the things I can't. That is important for you, too. Your awareness of your dog's normal aging processes will help you help her age well, and will help you know what is normal (and is, therefore, not something to get stressed about) and what is not normal (and is, therefore, something to ask your veterinarian about).

For gerontologists that deal with aging humans, there are many established measurements of physical health, cognitive health, and psychological health that they can use to assess their patients. For veterinarians that deal with aging dogs, there are no standardized measurements that are used, although efforts are now underway to establish some. A recent article in the *Journal of the American Veterinary Association* discussed the development of a working definition of healthy aging in dogs, and identified clinical methods for veterinarians to use to differentiate healthy aging from disease states.[1] You'd think that would be easy for us to do—but since the very definition of "health" is "the state of being free from illness or injury," it would seem that those of us who are older and have accrued a few age-related conditions would be, by that definition, considered unhealthy. However, that definition gets a little blurry when you consider that, if those conditions are not decreasing our quality of life and our ability to function in the ways we want to function, we should still be considered to be healthy, albeit aged, humans. That should be true for our dogs as well.

There are trends that you can expect to see as your dog passes from young adulthood into middle age and then into the senior years. The actual age in years when your dog qualifies for these labels varies and is, really, fairly arbitrary. I see so many dogs that live comfortably to their mid-teens that I have a hard time agreeing with the American Animal Hospital's designation of seven years as the age at which a dog is considered a "senior." Many of the seven-year-old dogs I see now will live another seven years—isn't seven only halfway along the aging continuum, and, therefore, by definition "middle-age"?

It is true, however, that what is the middle phase of chronological age and what is the geriatric phase depends on the breed and size of the dog since these factors influence how quickly a dog ages. Dogs that have a body weight of fifty pounds or more are classified as senior when they are six to eight years of age, and as geriatric when they are older than nine years of age. Dogs with a body weight of less than fifty pounds are considered senior at seven to ten years of age, and geriatric starting at eleven years of age. On average, an increase in body size of ten kilograms (twenty-two pounds) is associated with six months to one year of reduced lifespan. Currently, it is not understood why this is true— although there is one hint: in mice, evidence points to an influence by circulating levels of *insulin-like growth factor* (IGF-1). This term may actually sound familiar to you—this just happens to be the gene, described in chapter 3, that encodes for body size, which, since it is very prone to mutations, is responsible for the astounding variation between breeds in canine body size—and just might be responsible for the correlation between body size and longevity.

In addition to breed and size, there are other factors that influence aging rate in dogs; these include genetic makeup, exposure to injuries and disease, how effectively those injuries and diseases were treated, and nutritional state. As a general rule, dogs that are under five years of age are considered to be *young adults* (similar to humans under forty), dogs between five and nine years to be *middle-aged* (similar to humans between forty and sixty), dogs between nine and twelve years to be *senior* (similar to humans over sixty-six), and dogs over twelve to be *geriatric*.

Where is your dog on the adult/senior/geriatric spectrum? It's easiest to use the chronological definition, taking your dog's age, size, and breed into account, but, of course, your dog is an individual, with her own unique set of genetic, environmental, and lifestyle factors that influence her aging process. I suggest that you focus less on your dog's age in years, and focus more on how the years are, or are not, affecting your dog's ability to function in the way that you envisioned when you filled out your dog's job description at the end of chapter 1. This may change in subtle ways as time goes on, so as your dog ages, fill out a yearly performance evaluation and review the previous ones to identify trends. In addition, using the personality and behavior assessment tools in chapter 2 as well as your monthly physical exam checklists, you will also see how age is affecting, but not *afflicting*, your own individual dog.

General guidelines about what is or isn't healthy aging are only useful if you have a way to judge what optimal physical and behavioral health for your own dog has been in the context of your own lives, and that is only possible if you keep track of it over time. For example, if your dog has always jumped in the car, and suddenly can't, it means something different than if she could never jump in the car in the first place. Many of my clients are unaware of changes, such as hearing loss, in their dogs since they occur so gradually, until the hearing loss has gone past a certain threshold level when the dogs suddenly seem to have gone deaf—then they (the clients, not the dogs) get stressed about it and worry about some underlying disease. Hearing loss is normal as aging occurs—but it is in the "healthy aging" category, and one for which you can compensate if you are aware that it is happening. Helping your dog stay in the healthy aging portion of the continuum involves the use of your knowledge of her changes, and your ability to help her adjust to them, thus maintaining as much functionality as possible. There are some changes to expect, and the following information will keep you from being taken by surprise by them.

15

BEWARE THE CREEP

Definition of calorie: Tiny creatures that live in your closet that sew your clothes a little tighter each night. —Anonymous

Many battle with weight and know a few things about the equation related to calories consumed versus calories burned—if we eat too many calories, or burn too few, we gain weight; if we eat too few calories or burn too many (that never happens to me), we lose weight. We focus on the calories burned by activity, because that variable is within our control. But remember the hidden factor in the equation that many of us forget—our metabolic rate. You may remember that this is the rate at which our bodies burn calories to get the energy needed to maintain vital functions like breathing, pumping our hearts, circulating our blood, maintaining a normal body temperature, and keeping our brains alive and our internal organs functioning.

Part of what determines each individual's metabolic rate is lean body mass, or muscle mass. As a dog grows older, there is a reduction in maintenance energy requirements which has been estimated to be 20 percent, but may be higher—up to 50 percent! The primary reason for this is an age-related decrease in lean body mass with an accompanying increase in fat body mass. Loss of muscle is known as *sarcopenia* and occurs, in part, because there is a decrease in the number of muscle cells as well as a decrease in the size of the muscle cells themselves—this affects strength, stamina, and metabolic rate. Sarcopenia contributes to the other factors that cause weight gain, such as a decrease in activity and a consequent decrease in calorie use.

Dogs that have been spayed or neutered have an additional hidden factor that affects their metabolic rate and weight—the removal of the ovaries and the estrogen they produce, or the testes and the testosterone they produce, reduces the use of calories by 35 percent! It is definitely a good idea to spay and neuter dogs, despite this side effect, but many owners don't realize that they must compensate for this decrease in metabolic rate by feeding fewer calories and increasing activity over the life of their dogs. It's no wonder that so many dogs are overweight or even obese!

I notice that what I call "the weight creep" starts to happen at about the age of two or three years—people get used to feeding their one-year-old dogs a certain amount of food once they achieve adulthood, and then keep feeding that same amount through the years without taking into account how the calories from that food are being used. Dogs don't usually gain excessive weight between one and two years of age, since they are behaviorally and metabolically "teenagers"—and you know how teenagers can eat and not gain weight! But as they move further into adulthood, dogs gradually settle down a little, use fewer calories per year, lose a few muscle cells per year, and gain a few fat cells per year—until the weight creeps up and they are officially fat.

Remember to use the body condition scoring system shown in chapter 5 since this is the easiest way to see if the amount of fat your dog is carrying on her frame is becoming excessive. Weighing your dog regularly and watching how that correlates with your assessment of her body condition is especially important as your dog starts to age—this gives you an objective way to double-check your somewhat subjective body condition score and make sure you are on track.

Also, since lean muscle mass tends to decrease with increasing age, you need to monitor that as well, particularly because muscle mass has such an effect on not only the metabolic rate but also strength and stamina. In fact, an increase in fat and a decrease in muscle mass can cancel each other out and make the weight and body condition score stay the same—unless you pay attention to certain areas.

One of the areas where you can notice loss of muscle mass is on the forehead area, above the eyes up to an imaginary line that runs between both ears. This area should be slightly rounded, but, if muscle mass is being lost, it can look flat or even concave. Other areas to watch are over the shoulder blades, along the backbone, and above the hips—if the bones are sticking out there, your dog may be losing muscle mass or losing too much weight. Fat gain and muscle loss do not occur in every dog; however, many geriatric dogs will lose weight as they grow older—this may be related to their breed, but could be the result of an undiagnosed or uncontrolled age-related disease. Paying attention to weight, body condition, and muscle mass will allow you to intervene by decreasing calorie intake and increasing activity if the fat mass is going up and the muscle mass is going down, or to consult your veterinarian to see if any diagnostic tests are needed if the fat mass and the muscle mass are both going down.

As your dog's chef, personal trainer, and home health-care provider, you can offset these changes, if you detect them early. Choosing a different diet, and modifying activity to burn calories and build strength are simple lifestyle fixes that those of us who have reached middle age must do to maintain good body condition—and it's really not all that hard to do the same for our dogs.

Your choice of food for your dog is probably the biggest part of this, but it can be difficult to know what food to choose for an aging dog. Many foods are formulated specifically for "senior" dogs, and they can be a good choice, but, in my opinion, not an absolutely necessary one. Senior diets tend to have fewer calories, higher amounts of fiber, lower amounts of protein, and frequently contain dietary supplements to improve joint health. Lowering the calories in food is often appropriate for senior dogs, but you can easily find other low-calorie foods. By reading the labels or checking out the food's website, you can usually find the number of calories that a food contains.

As for protein content, senior dogs actually need a higher, not lower, amount of protein to maintain their muscle mass. Senior diets were originally designed to have lower amounts of protein because it was thought that, since older dogs are more likely to have kidney problems, and a lower protein diet is recommended for dogs with kidney dysfunction, kidney problems could then be prevented by the use of a low protein diet early in the senior years. This theory has since been disproven—in fact, in older dogs, there is increased protein metabolism and decreased protein synthesis, but protein absorption stays the same. Given these changes, having adequate protein content in the diet is more important as age increases. Senior diets also have lower phosphorus and sodium levels since these restrictions can be helpful in dogs with kidney disease—but, again, these restrictions will not prevent kidney disease. It is important to note, however, that senior diets are not properly balanced in protein, phosphorus, and sodium for those dogs that actually *do* have kidney disease, and cannot be substituted for prescription diets designed for those patients.

As for the joint supplements that are in senior diets, they are potentially very helpful—but it is better to give them to your dog separately. The correct supplement dose is dependent on a dog's weight, but the amount of the supplement that a dog gets out of a diet is dependent on how much that dog eats—and some dogs of the same weight eat more or less than others, and, therefore, may not be getting the right dose.

So, ultimately, senior diets are fine to use, although not truly necessary, but check the label for calorie and protein content. Try to choose one that contains the right number of calories for your dog's needs as time goes on and her weight changes along with an increasing protein content to match her increasing age.

As long as we are talking about food we might as well talk about digestion. As dogs get older, there are changes that occur in the gastrointestinal tract—a decrease in salivary and gastric acid secretion, a reduction in the rate at which food moves from the stomach into the small intestine, a reduction of the absorptive surfaces of the small intestine, a decrease in the peristaltic movements of the large intestine, and a change in the composition of the "gut microbiota" (the vast population of trillions of different bacteria that live in our intestine throughout our lives). However, despite these changes, dogs appear to continue to digest quite efficiently as they age and don't require adjustments in food digestibility. The decrease in how fast the stomach empties makes aging humans feel full faster and longer, and this may be true for dogs as well—and you can take advantage of this as you are adjusting calorie intake for your aging dog.

The addition of fiber into the diet can make it easier for an older dog, especially those with some arthritis in the back legs, to pass stools. The fiber cannot only make the stools easier to pass, but can also support a healthy bacterial population.

The gut microbiota is currently an area of intense research. There is some evidence that the composition of the bacterial population plays a role not only in digestive health, but also in body-wide health and affects inflammation, immunity, weight control—even mood. Probiotics are supplements that contain live microorganisms that, when composed of certain bacterial strains administered in adequate amounts, can have specific health benefits. Exactly how this occurs is still being evaluated, and this can make recommendations about the use of probiotics in both humans and dogs difficult. The gut microbiota does appear to evolve throughout life, and is affected by diet, drug use, the environment—and aging. It is thought that the change in the bacterial composition that occurs with advancing age may play a role in age-related deterioration of the immune system.[1] The use of probiotics may help counteract this process, and although more research will be needed to know exactly which strains of bacteria are effective for different health benefits, I would recommend the use of probiotics for dogs of any age with recurrent digestive problems, such as diarrhea, and would also recommend their use in older dogs, for the reasons mentioned earlier. The use of probiotics appears to be safe and many forms are available—but buyer beware—there have been problems with the reliability of some products, with some being tested and found to have no live organisms. Three have been found to contain the quantity and type of organisms on the label, and I would recommend choosing from one of the following:

Proviable-DC (nutramaxlabs.com)
FortiFlora (purina.com)
Prostora (iams.com)

As always, check with your veterinarian to see if probiotic supplementation is appropriate for your own dog.

16

SHIFTING SENSES

Question: Why do ophthalmologists live so long? Answer: Because they dilate. —Favorite joke told by my father, an ophthalmologist

Your dog's ability to interact with her world, and with you, is largely dependent on her five senses. All five of these senses change significantly with increasing age, and, whereas your dog probably has no awareness of these changes or the reasons for them, she will be shaped by them over time. Her mobility, behavior, appetite, and sleep will be altered, her way of relating to you will be different, and this, in turn, will change how you will relate to her. The reason this is so important is that many people are not aware that these behavioral changes are a logical outcome of normal age-related sensory changes, and often misunderstand their dog's changed behavior—sometimes attributing other causes that they then try, and fail, to correct. Is a dog that no longer responds to the command "Come" being defiant, or is she losing her hearing? Is a dog that can't catch a treat out of the air anymore getting senile, or is her vision changing?

Many of the same sensory changes also occur in people, and we anticipate them, understand them, and compensate for them without even thinking about it. Anyone who has had an aging parent or grandparent realizes that, if that person doesn't turn around when spoken to, it's due to poor hearing, not lack of caring or attention. Most of us would then automatically try to adjust for the hearing loss by getting in front of that person to be seen, and, therefore, noticed. We all know what is happening, because our aging human counterparts tell us what it's like, and we all know that it will also happen to us someday. Do declines in hearing, vision, and mobility keep us humans from enjoying the world as we go through our golden years? No! We have hearing aids, glasses, canes, walkers, and many, many assistive devices that allow us to compensate for those changes—and not give in to them. Reductions in hearing, vision, and mobility shouldn't keep your dog from enjoying the world either—especially since she has a great built-in assistive device to help her compensate—you! Your dog can't tell you what it is like to be an aging dog, but I can! Then you can use your new caninomorphic powers to, first, imagine how it feels to be your aging dog and, second, think of ways you can help her adjust to her sensory changes. This knowledge will help you make adjustments in your home, your lifestyle, and even your attitude, and will make her world safe and comfortable, which will, in turn, allow her to continue to be the unique individual you picked out all those years ago.

VISION

Let's go from the outside of the eye to the inside, like we did before:

Lids, Globe, and Muscles

- Since the skin, cartilage, and muscles thin with age, the lids of the aging dog do not open as widely as they used to. In addition, there is a change in the way the eyeball, or globe, sits in the socket, often due to a decrease in the amount of fat behind the eye, and the globe appears to be more sunken into the socket—this also causes the lids to be closer together.
- The muscles that govern eyeball movement diminish in strength, and decrease how far the eyes can rotate to look side-to-side or up and down. All of these things combine to decrease some peripheral vision and limit the size of the visual field. The visual field refers to the total area in which objects can be seen while the eyes are focused on a central point.
- It's common for dogs, as they age, to develop small tumors on the edge of the eyelids, and these can block a little vision. Most of these are noncancerous, but some can grow large, and there are a few that

are cancerous. Please see your veterinarian if you notice any bumps on your dog's eyelids to see if they should be removed.

Cornea

- The clarity of the outer coating of the eye is dependent, in part, on moisture provided by the tear-producing *lacrimal glands*, located in the eyelids. Tear production tends to go down as age goes up, probably due to age-related degeneration in the lacrimal glands. You may notice that your dog's eyes are not as shiny as they once were since there is less moisture on and in the corneas to reflect light. The dryness of the cornea scatters some of the light hitting it, and the transmission of light through the drier corneas becomes less efficient than it used to be.
- The density of cells of the cornea decreases with age, and so does the thickness of the cornea. In turn, the sensitivity of the cornea becomes diminished and the ability of the older dog to protect her eyes from injury may be impaired, while at the same time, the ability of the cornea to repair itself after injury may also be reduced.
- There is a change in corneal contour that occurs with age: this changes how the cornea bends the light that passes through it to get to the lens and retina. The cornea develops a slightly different surface curvature in one direction from the other—instead of being even and smooth in all directions, the surface may have some areas that are flatter or steeper. This is known as astigmatism, and causes distortion of the light rays as they pass through the cornea, which blurs vision slightly at all distances.

Iris and Pupil

- The iris becomes thinner and your dog's eye color may shift a little due to the difference in the way light bounces off the iris. This iris atrophy may cause irregularity of the edges of the pupillary slit.
- The pupil itself will be slightly smaller, and will not open up as far to admit more light in dim conditions.
- The speed at which the pupil can grow larger or smaller in response to ambient light is reduced, and your dog may have trouble adjusting

to sudden lighting changes, such as going out into bright sunlight or moving from a dark room to a room that has bright lights or a shiny floor.

Lens

The lens goes through several important age-related changes:

- It becomes less flexible with age, because the outer coating, the lens capsule, becomes less elastic, and the fibers within the lens itself become more compacted. This, combined with decreased strength of the ciliary body (the pulleys attached to the edges of the lens which change its shape) impairs the ability of the lens to change shape in order to focus an image on the back of the eye. The image of objects that are far away needs less bending to bring it into focus, whereas the image of objects that are close, which seem larger, needs more bending by thicker lenses to bring it into focus. If the lens can't become thicker, objects that are close appear blurry while objects that are far away are still sharp. When this happens to humans, we simply (albeit reluctantly) buy reading glasses to compensate.

  Close vision is less important to the canine species, and is already somewhat blurry because lenses of dogs are stiff to begin with, but this aging change makes it even blurrier—and it can manifest itself in unexpected ways in the lives of our pet dogs. If you see an older dog hesitating to jump up on furniture or into the car, you might think that the hesitation is due to arthritis. It may be due, in part, to that, but it can also be due to the dog's inability to see the edge of the seat, and that hesitation may be occurring because the dog is simply trying to figure out how high or how far to jump. Many older dogs will pause at the top or bottom of a stairway—this may be because they can't really discern the edge of the first step, or see the difference between the first step and the series of steps afterward. Try looking down a long stairway in dim light through a plastic food storage bag, and imagine taking that first step without really seeing it—you'd be afraid of falling, too!

- As the lens ages, it continues to produce lens fibers, and the older fibers become more and more compressed as the new ones accumulate. This causes increased lens density, and appears as a bluish-gray haziness to the lens, called *nuclear sclerosis* or *lenticular sclerosis*, which many people mistake as cataracts. Cataracts are different—those occur when protein clumps form within the lens, and as they develop, they significantly impair light transmission through those areas. When fully formed, they appear as bright white structures behind the pupil and no light can get through them so that vision is blocked. Nuclear sclerosis commonly starts around the age of six to seven years, and does not, in itself, impair vision, although the process that causes it also causes the stiffness of the lens, which interferes with near vision.
- Cataracts are an almost inevitable consequence of aging in humans and are common in geriatric dogs as well. Age-related cataracts rarely progress to the fully formed, totally opaque phase, although this can happen in certain conditions, such as uncontrolled diabetes, but the opacities in the lenses do significantly interfere with vision as they accumulate over time. One study looked at the age at which dogs developed cataracts and found it to be dependent on the dog's breed, with larger dogs developing them earlier than smaller ones.[1] For all the dogs studied, 50 percent had developed age-related cataracts between the ages of six and twelve years, and 100 percent of those over 13.5 years had developed cataracts. In terms of longevity, it was estimated that cataracts occur when dogs have reached 68–85 percent of total lifespan. One study that looked at the use of age-related cataracts as a biomarker for longevity, using the theory that cataracts are due to the accumulation of reactive oxygen species within the cells, found a correlation between cataracts and breed- and size-related longevity—small-breed dogs (who generally have greater longevity) developed cataracts at a later age than large-breed dogs.[2]
- All the factors that promote cataract formation in dogs are unknown, but there are two factors that promote them in humans that may be relevant to dogs. These are ultraviolet light and dehydration—both of which are under your control. For example, controlling long-term exposure to UV light and ensuring adequate

water intake while your dog participates in outdoor activities is up to you, and so is your choice of a diet or the use of supplements that contain antioxidants to combat the accumulation of reactive oxygen species in the lenses. Fortunately, age-related cataracts are unlikely to progress to the point that your dog will become blind, but they will cause the vision to be increasingly blurred. In age-related cataracts, the lenses will gradually become cloudier, and will also become slightly yellower—this means that the lens will act as a filter for light of shorter wavelengths, which correspond to the colors of purple for humans and blue for dogs, making these colors appear dull or gray.

- Those with cataracts have more difficulty with vision at night and are more sensitive to light and glare, and, at least for people, "halos" appear around lights.

Retina

- The cells within the retina undergo many changes with increasing age—the cells change in their shape and volume, their numbers decrease, their pigments increase, old cells aren't removed, the blood supply to the retina diminishes, and the numbers of nerve cells carrying information to the brain are decreased.
- Photoreceptor cells are lost as the retina ages, and this causes the retina to become thinner, especially at the periphery. Some of the cells that remain develop an abnormal orientation within the retina, so that incoming light, traveling on a straight axis, hits those cells in the retina at a different angle than before, and impairs the ability of those cells to respond to that light. These cells will, however, respond to light that has been scattered by things like dried-out corneas, cloudy lenses and floaters, which is why glare interferes with the vision in older individuals more than younger ones. Some light also is bounced around on the inside of the eye by the tapetum (that reflective coating over part of the retina) and this may create more light scatter.
- The loss of the cone photoreceptors in the aging canine retina was found to be greater than the loss of rod receptors in one study and was 30 percent and 15 percent, respectively.[3] Since dogs have more rods than cones, the loss of rods has a disproportionately high impact

on vision for them and would have its greatest effect in dim lighting conditions and in the detection of objects in the edges of the visual field. Loss of cones affects both visual detail and color discrimination, meaning that higher intensities of color are needed for visual perception to occur.

For both species, the impairment of color discrimination causes significant changes in the quality of lives of aging individuals—unless some compensations are made. The need for higher color intensity causes poor contrast sensitivity, which makes the detection of the edges of objects, such as stairs, difficult. Contrast sensitivity is a measurement of the smallest amount of contrast that can be perceived—good contrast sensitivity means that a person (or dog) can distinguish between two things with little difference in intensity while those with increasingly poor contrast sensitivity need an increasingly large difference in intensities to distinguish between those things. This is also related to the size of the objects—those with poor contrast sensitivity have less of a problem when the objects of similar intensity are large. For aging people, it can be difficult to read if the printed letters are of similar intensity to the background, such as black letters on a gray background, and high-contrast text, with black letters on a white background, is easier to read.

For aging dogs, it can be difficult to see the edges of individual steps on a staircase as there is little contrast between them. Marking the edges of steps with black electrical tape or placing self-adhesive abrasive tape strips (available at hardware stores) on wooden steps can help increase your older dog's sense of security, as well as her safety, when she goes down a flight of stairs. Try to look around your home, and your yard, and see if you can spot areas that have poor contrast, but, while you are doing so, remember that your dog has fewer cones, so he also sees the colors of the world in a less saturated way—even before aging desaturates the world even more.

Look at your environment through caninomorphic lenses: the colors that you see as violet or bluish-purple are probably seen as some shade of blue; the colors you see as greenish-yellow, yellow, and red are probably seen as yellow; the colors you see as green-blue are probably seen as some shade of gray. If, in your mind's eye, you can take out lots of color, take out lots of intensity, and then also take out the contrast as you look around your dog's environment, you might be able to "see" lots of things your dog might trip over or be confused by, and then be able to modify to make it easier for her.

While you're at it, look at yourself in the mirror—many features within the human face are of low contrast, especially the nose and lips. Your dog, as she gets older, may not be able to read your facial expression or may not even recognize you at all sometimes—but don't be offended—she still cares about you! Many owners use facial expression, among other body language cues, along with words to communicate with their dogs without even realizing it. When your dog's vision becomes blurred with aging, your face probably looks like those people on TV that want to keep their identities hidden during interviews, so the camera puts a blurry patch over just the person's face—this, to me is a little disconcerting since I can't read the person's emotions or see the mouth and lips move during speech. Imagine your dog looking at you with that kind of blurring on your face—it would probably hide your identity and emotions, too—at least until she was able to use her olfactory superpower to identify you! Having the lights on to better illuminate your face will help, and so will the use of exaggerated facial expressions or gestures.

Using those hand signals you taught your dog all those years ago, in an especially dramatic way, will also aid in keeping the lines of communication open between the two of you. Remember that her field of vision is narrower than it used to be. Make sure you are in the center of her visual field when getting her attention or using the hand signals, and when you play ball or Frisbee with her, throw things a little more into the center of her field of vision rather than on the edges so she will detect the movement. Fine detail discrimination is not needed for most games, but paying attention to the contrast of the toy will be necessary as your dog's contrast sensitivity will lessen with age.

Also, pay attention to what you wear and how much contrast your clothes have, too—if you wear a gray sweatshirt for an off-leash walk in the woods in the winter, you may be practically invisible, so wear black in those surroundings. For green surroundings, which will appear a pale grayish-brownish-yellow, black or a deep, bright blue would be a good look for you—at least as far as your dog is concerned! Under most circumstances, especially at home, your dog's excellent sense of smell will make up for your dog's decrease in visual acuity—but, in unfamiliar surroundings, or outside, where she may be less able to track you by scent, you will need to compensate for it on her behalf to keep her safe and to make her feel secure—luckily, you have the cognitive abilities and, now, the knowledge she lacks.

17

TURN UP THE VOLUME

Kindness is the language that the deaf can hear and the blind can
see. —Mark Twain

Age-related hearing loss is known as *presbycusis* and is characterized
by gradual and progressive loss of hearing in both ears over many years.
The cause of presbycusis may really be a combination of degenerative
changes related to aging plus the cumulative effects of other insults to
the hearing apparatus over the lifetime of an individual. The many
molecular, biochemical, and physiologic changes associated with the
aging process in other parts of the body also appear to contribute to
presbycusis. Other factors that contribute to hearing loss over time in
humans are: chronic noise exposure, drugs, or chemicals that directly
damage the inner ear (certain antibiotics, chemotherapy drugs, heavy
metals), infections, smoking, high blood pressure, diabetes, vascular
disease, immunologic disorders, genetic factors, and hormones. Some
of these same factors have also been shown to contribute to the development of presbycusis in dogs.

Let's review some of the anatomy of the hearing apparatus (don't
worry—this will be brief). The ear can be divided into three anatomic
areas: the external ear, middle ear, and inner ear. The external ear
includes the pinna and the external ear canal, which direct sounds to
the middle ear; this area includes the tympanic membrane, tympanic
cavity, the three ear bones (ossicles), and the eustachian tube. The
inner ear contains the organ of hearing, the cochlea, and the organ of
balance, the vestibular system; both of these translate the motion of

fluid around hair cells (from either sound or head acceleration) into nerve signals. Within the inner ear, the blood vessels of the stria vascularis produce the fluid (or endolymph) for the scala media, which is one of three fluid-filled compartments within the cochlea. The nerve signals stimulated by the hair cells and their surrounding fluid enter the spiral ganglion and are then carried to the brain by the vestibulocochlear (eighth) cranial nerve. Hearing loss, in general, is classified into two main types:

- *Sensorineural*—involving the inner ear, cochlea, or the auditory nerve.
- *Conductive*—involving anything that limits the amount of sound that gets to the inner ear. Examples include debris in the outer ear canal, fluid in the middle ear, thickening of the eardrum, or a lack of movement of the small bones of the ear.

Presbycusis is a type of sensorineural hearing loss—and that is what we will be focusing on in this section—but it is important to be aware that, as your dog gets older, anything that causes a decrease in conductive hearing will be superimposed on age-related hearing loss and will magnify the degree of hearing loss. Some of the causes of conductive hearing loss can be eliminated or at least lessened, so you may be able to preserve some of your dog's hearing if you and your vet pay attention to them. In dogs, a seven-year longitudinal study found that auditory acuity started to decline at eight to ten years of age, and the mid- to high-range frequencies of 8–32 kHz were affected first.[1] The hearing loss was progressive and eventually spanned the entire frequency range. Two other studies on dogs found that all of the dogs in the study had hearing loss by the age of twelve years and that structural changes were most prominent at that age, with many of them being most severe at the base of the cochlea, which corresponds to the area that detects mid- to high-frequency sounds.[2]

What does the loss of hearing mean for humans? People with hearing loss describe a sense of isolation, and the onset of deafness is associated with poorer physical health, decreased physical activity, and depression. What does hearing loss mean for dogs? It is hard to know how a dog feels when the hearing decreases; humans have the ability to understand what is happening as they lose their hearing, and have many ways of compensating for it, yet they still have difficulties adjusting to it.

I don't know if dogs go through these same emotions as they lose their hearing—after all, dogs probably don't have the cognitive abilities needed to reflect upon this change, but they do react to it, and they can behave differently as a result. Your ability to understand what it might be like for your dog to lose her hearing will help you help her negotiate her world. Since the hearing changes that occur with age appear similar in humans and dogs, we can safely extrapolate some of what we know about humans to our dogs.

Humans with presbycusis describe that sounds often seem less clear and lower in volume. This is because the frequencies most affected by presbycusis are those above 2 kHz; then, over time, the high frequencies continue to drop, and the mid and low frequencies (0.5 to 2 kHz), which are important in human speech, become progressively involved. The low and mid frequencies of human speech are the areas that carry the majority of energy of the sound wave and include most of the vowel sounds in words. The high frequencies, however, carry the consonant sounds and the majority of the information in speech. These consonant sounds tend to be not only high pitched, but also soft, which makes them particularly difficult for patients with presbycusis to hear. As a result of this hearing loss pattern, patients with high-frequency hearing loss will often report being able to hear when someone is speaking (because of the louder, low-frequency vowels), but not being able to understand what is being said (because of the loss of consonant information), and that high-pitched sounds such as "s" and "th" are difficult to hear and tell apart. They will describe that a man's voice is easier to hear than the higher pitches of a woman's voice, or that they can't hear the chirping of a bird, but can hear the sound of an approaching truck.

The missing high frequencies also cause people with presbycusis to have a greater decline in hearing while in an environment that has even a small amount of background noise, because it is the high frequencies that are essential to allow the inner ear to focus on sounds of particular interest and pick out those sounds from competing ambient noise. People with presbycusis also have a decreased ability to tolerate sudden, loud noises, and many report a ringing, roaring, or hissing sound in one or both ears, known as tinnitus.

Age-related changes to another part of the inner ear, the labyrinth, which is called *presbyastasis*, causes problems with balance and, in a more extreme form, vertigo—which is when the person, or dog, feels as if her body is spinning in space or that the world is whirling around her body. Presbyastasis can cause falls and is even worse if that individual has any problems with her vision, has stiff joints, or has numb feet, since vision and touch help the brain know where the body is in relationship to the physical surroundings.

There is no common grading system for hearing loss in dogs, as there is in humans—but what is important for dog owners to know is how their dogs hear in their home environment—whether or not their dogs hear their voices, understand their commands, hear the doorbell, or hear intruders. Many dogs with hearing impairment can seem less responsive, overly sleepy, and more inattentive, and, for those that are getting older, it is hard for their owners to tell the difference between age-related hearing loss and age-related cognitive dysfunction or dementia. It would be useful to have a grading system for owners to assess their dog's hearing in the home setting, particularly over time as their dogs age.

In an attempt to establish a hearing impairment grading system, a questionnaire was devised for use by owners of dogs that were being referred for evaluation of chronic middle ear infections.[3] I think it useful for you to use this questionnaire on an ongoing basis as your dog becomes older and enters the years when age-related hearing loss can begin. After all, the point of presenting the information in this book is to give you the tools to be aware of the changes happening in your dog so you can do what you can to prevent them or at least help compensate for them. I have included this questionnaire as a tool for intermittent assessment of your dog's hearing—you could do this with your monthly physical exams, or perhaps less often, such as every two to three months. Record the results over time, since hearing loss is gradual and subtle, and your repeated hearing assessments should be consistent with that usual trend. If, however, based on your ongoing hearing assessments, your dog has mild hearing impairment and then it is suddenly profound, you should have her evaluated for causes of conductive hearing loss that superimposed on the ongoing age-related hearing loss. Presbycusis may not be reversible but conductive hearing loss can be, and improvement in your dog's hearing could be as simple as taking the wax out of her ears or curing an ear infection!

This questionnaire was designed to evaluate a dog's response to common noises in the home and to noises in which most dogs would take an interest. The owners were asked to answer yes or no to the following eight questions:

1. Do you think your dog hears well?
2. Does your dog hear a knock at the door or hear the doorbell?
3. Does your dog hear cars as they pull into the drive?
4. Does your dog hear a car door slam in the driveway?
5. Does your dog bark more loudly than she used to? (some dogs never bark, so eliminate this question if that is true for your dog)
6. Does your dog sleep soundly? (that is, fail to stir while asleep when you enter the room)
7. If you stand behind your dog, does she hear you when you clap your hands?
8. If you stand behind your dog, does she hear you when you whisper her name?

Every two "yes" answers are assigned one point; one point corresponds with mild hearing impairment, two points corresponds with moderate hearing impairment, three points corresponds with severe hearing impairment, and four points corresponds with profound impairment. For your reference, the estimated loudness measures for common environmental sounds are:

- whisper: 20 dB
- normal conversational speech: 50–65 dB
- heavy traffic: 80 dB
- thunderclap: 120 dB

You can use these loudness measures to estimate your dog's degree of hearing loss at home, and to roughly know how much to modify the loudness of your voice for her to hear. Of course, you won't easily measure the decibel level of your own voice (although there is an app for that!), but you can see from the measures in the previous list that normal conversational speech is about three times louder than a whisper. Experimenting with the intensity of your voice to see when she hears you, while she is not looking at you, can be helpful.

Now you know how to monitor hearing loss in your dog—but you also need to know some ways to prevent it. Presbycusis is the result of the cumulative effects of heredity, disease, noise, and agents toxic to the hearing apparatus. Although you can't do anything about your dog's heredity, you may be able to modify some of the other factors.

One of the most preventable causes of hearing loss is to reduce repeated or constant exposure to loud noises. Excessive noise, compounded over time, can ultimately affect the degree of presbycusis that your dog develops. The mechanism by which excessive noise induces hearing loss includes direct mechanical damage of cochlear structures and metabolic overload in those structures, due to overstimulation. There are protective reflexes in the middle ear where muscles contract in response to loud sounds, and this can decrease the amount of sound that reaches the middle ear, but the reflexes are too slow for sharp, sudden loud sounds, such as gunfire, and don't protect well against these types of sounds. Extremely loud sounds (over 120–155 dB) can damage the eardrum and the ossicles. In general, except for these types of percussive sounds, the degree of structural damage is related to both the intensity of the sound as well as the duration of the sound.

Noise-induced hearing loss can be temporary or permanent—permanent hearing loss occurs when there is damage to the hair cells of the organ of Corti. Studies in humans and animals have shown that there are two periods of increased susceptibility to noise exposure—one is early in life (during adolescence and early adulthood), and the other is later in life; in mice, early noise exposure, even of short duration, can trigger a progressive loss of hearing much later in life.

What kind of noises could your dog encounter that could damage her hearing? Certain noises like gunfire or explosions would be obvious candidates, but for the nonhunting owners out there, there are plenty of other sounds around that can do it—lawn mowers, leaf-blowers, woodworking equipment, shop vacs, snowmobiles, motorcycles, loud music—even noise in boarding kennels.

One study examined measured noise levels in a laboratory kennel and in an animal shelter, and also measured the hearing of the dogs at forty-eight hours, three months, and six months after arrival.[4] The noise levels from the barking dogs in an environment with bare concrete walls were measured at between 100 and 108 dB and, at the end of six months, all dogs had a measurable change in hearing. Think of how much hearing damage your dog could have at the kennel during your usual vacations—this means you need to only board your dog in a kennel or use daycare facilities that have good noise abatement strategies, such as acoustic tile and other sound-dampening materials.

As for the other potential sources of noise-related hearing damage for your dog, be careful how loud you play your stereo in your car and keep your dog inside your house when you are doing work in the yard or in the woodshop. You can actually measure the decibel level of your own environment and the noise produced by whatever activities you enjoy with one of the many apps available for that purpose. Once you download one of those apps, stick your smartphone out the window while your car is going fifty-five miles per hour—you might think twice about letting your dog stick her head out once you realize how loud the rushing air is! All in all, short of putting protective ear muffs on your dog (none are currently available anyway), preventing exposure to loud noise is your best bet to prevent noise-induced hearing damage in your dog (and yourself).

Another way to prevent hearing loss in your dog is to be aware of substances that can damage the hearing apparatus—these are known as ototoxins. More than 180 drugs and chemicals have been found to be toxic to both of the organs in the inner ear, the cochlea and the vestibular apparatus, and can, therefore, damage the hearing or the balance. Toxins can directly damage the hair cells or indirectly damage the stria vascularis. The effects can be temporary or permanent, can result from brief or long-term exposures, can be through direct contact (via diffusion through the middle ear) or through the bloodstream. If there is preexisting noise-induced hearing damage or presbycusis, the ototoxic effects can become worse.

Common drugs that can be ototoxic include certain antibiotics (such as gentamycin and tobramycin), loop diuretics (such as furosemide, a.k.a. Lasix), salicylates (such as aspirin), and chemotherapy agents (cisplatin and carboplatin). Gentamycin is commonly found in ear medications used to treat ear infections of the external ear canal (otitis externa) because it is very effective and relatively inexpensive. It is a very useful and effective antibiotic and its use is often justifiable despite its unpredictable potential to damage the hearing apparatus, especially since chronic ear infections can also damage hearing. Please discuss its use for your dog's ear infections with your veterinarian.

Remember that anything that is put into the external ear canal will create some conductive hearing loss, which will last for as long as the substance is in there, so don't panic if your dog doesn't hear you as well as usual after being treated for an ear infection. This will be temporary—the hearing loss induced by some of the other drugs, such as furosemide and aspirin, is also reversible.

There are a number of environmental chemicals and heavy metals that have been associated with hearing or balance problems in humans—since we share our environment with our dogs, there is no reason to think these same chemicals won't cause the same problem in our dogs. These include: mercury, lead, toluene, carbon disulfide, trichloroethylene, xylene, butyl nitrate, carbon monoxide, styrene, hexane, and manganese. You may not know how much of these things are in your own environment—hopefully very little—but avoid taking your dogs to places or letting her swim in, or drink out of, water where she might encounter those pollutants. Many streams and ponds in urban and what are now suburban areas may look clean, but are heavily polluted from former factories at that site, or farms upstream, so check with local environmental authorities about water pollution in your area.

What else can you do to protect your dog from hearing loss? Since age-related hearing loss is thought to be related to cellular degeneration due to exposure to oxidative products of metabolism (i.e., reactive oxygen species) studies have tested the effects of antioxidants on the aging inner ear. These found that providing either a diet or supplements that are rich in antioxidants resulted in less degeneration to the inner ear as dogs got older. For the dogs studied, dietary supplementation during the last 25 percent of the lifespan, using fruits, vegetables, antioxidants, and mitochondrial cofactors reduced the magnitude of cochlear cell loss. General diet and supplement recommendations will be presented later in this book.

What might dogs with presbycusis describe if they could? Well, it's time, once again, for a little caninomorphism! Based on the information presented earlier, you can now put yourself in your dog's shoes (or ears) and imagine how she might feel as she experiences gradual hearing loss, without understanding that it is even happening or why. If you can't hear sound as well, especially in the high frequencies, you would not notice the small sounds that you used to hear even while asleep. You would then fall deeper asleep than usual and wouldn't hear things like a car approaching or keys rattling in the door, and might not be at the door ready to joyfully greet someone who just came home. You might not even notice approaching footsteps and be extremely startled by a gentle touch on your back—you might, uncharacteristically, snarl or snap because, after all, you, as a dog, don't know if that touch is from someone who sees you as a friend or a food source. Then, say, you are home alone in a room in your home, and can't hear anything—would you know if your family was home, perhaps just in another room, or away from the house? Might you then start to seek our other forms of contact—olfactory, visual, tactile—by being clingy when your family is home or by wandering around looking for them when your family isn't?

Think about those forms of communication that your people are always using—called speech and language—that you used to understand and found so important in order to know what they wanted. Would words like "sit" and "stay," and even "no" or "good girl" sound the same, and would you respond to them the same way if you didn't recognize them anymore? After all, you can't hear high-frequency, low-volume consonants (like "z," "v," "m," "n," "d," "b") anymore, and, even if your low-frequency sensitivity is still there (for a while), you can hear your people talking, you won't understand what they are saying anymore. Would you seem indifferent or disobedient to your people? Would you be frustrated or anxious if you were really, really trying to please them but couldn't figure out what they wanted? The inability to hear the sounds and process them into language wouldn't be so bad if you could just hear all those high-pitched, baby talk sounds that used to give you some clue about the emotional content of the speech—is your person happy or sad, pleased or displeased? Maybe you could get a little information from your vision, but—oh yes—your fine visual discrimination ain't what it used to be! Even with specific areas in your canine brain that are devoted to making sense of vocalizations and that are attuned to their emotional content, it would be hard for your brain to perform those functions if you can't hear some or all of those sounds. Remember humans selected you for your ability to hear and understand what they were saying—wouldn't you find it hard not to be spoken to anymore, when you know you are supposed to be listening?

So, you can go back to being a human now—and use your own higher cognitive function to figure out how to make things easier for your dog over the next few years. This is the time to remember to practice your hand signals with your dog (see chapter 12). They can be crucial in communicating with her when she can't hear some of the sounds of your speech and can't put them together to understand the spoken language you use. Build the foundation of communication with your older dog while you have a younger dog, and keep practicing the signs. It doesn't really matter what gestures you make and what words you tie them with—they can be as unique as the two of you are—but try to create a good vocabulary using big gestures. In particular, ingrain the signals for "watch me" and "good dog" to get her accustomed to using her eyes in addition to her ears to gain communication from you, and keep practicing the hand signals for "sit," "stay," "down," and "come"— these will form the foundation of some physical therapy exercises that you will do when your dog is older and that are described at howtoage-proofyourdog.com.

Make sure you teach her some signals with some emotional content, too—your dog needs to know how you are feeling as well as what you are saying, and, as a dog that has an instinctual need to get that feedback, she will be anxious if you don't give it to her. Use exaggerated facial expressions to go along with whatever emotion you are trying to convey—see if you can translate that high baby-talk voice you've used since she was a puppy into a facial expression! Tie the positive content with tactile praise—petting or stroking—since, as you know, dogs prefer that to verbal praise. Over her lifetime, intermittently reinforce her accurate performance of the hand signals to keep her knowledge fresh and her associations with them positive.

How else to compensate for your dog's presbycusis? Remember she may not hear you when you come in the room, if she is asleep—so stomp on the floor on your way in or make some other loud sounds, preferably low-pitched, to warn her of your presence, so she won't be so startled. When you play with her, use very, very loud squeaky toys—for a long while, she will still hear high frequencies if they are made loud enough. When you use your voice, try to either increase the loudness level of your higher pitched vocalizations, or start to use lower frequencies when you talk to her. Remember that, when you try to communicate at a distance, low-pitched sounds will carry better than high-pitched ones, although you can raise the loudness level of higher-pitched vocalizations by singing them. This will come in handy at the park or somewhere else if your dog is off-leash—although it may make bystanders laugh! While she is off-leash and at a great distance, you can also use a sports whistle or even a brief toot on an air horn to get her attention so she can see your hand gestures. Practice that in a contained area at first, and follow that very loud, unfamiliar sound with a positive reinforcement (the "good dog gesture") the first few times you use it, but, since some dogs that lose their hearing become overly sensitive to loud sounds, if it startles your dog too much, just use your voice.

So far, we have focused mainly on the age-, noise-, and toxin-related damage to the hearing portion of the inner ear, the cochlea. The other inner ear organ, the labyrinth, is the one that governs the sense of balance, and that can be damaged by those same factors. The same preventative techniques apply, but the manifestation of this change will be very different. The loss of balance can be gradual, mild, and subtle and may show itself in some unsteadiness on slick surfaces, going up or down stairs, jumping up on furniture and in cars, difficulty staying up-right while riding in the bouncy car. Take care to support your dog's body under these circumstances if she seems wobbly—sometimes, just a hand on her back or sides will do the trick, and, sometimes, a harness that you can grasp from over her back will help. This would be equiva-lent to a walker or cane for some people who aren't paralyzed, just unsteady, and need just another way to know where their bodies are in space and how to counter the false signals their equilibrium monitors in their inner ears are sending their brains.

Helping your dog stay on surfaces with good traction, or supplying good traction to her, will help prevent falls as her feet may slip more easily as she tries to maintain her balance. Putting carpet runners on tile or wooden floors will give her secure footing, and, if there is contrast with the underlying floor color, can even look like a kind of "runway" to guide her. If runners aren't an option, there are booties that you can get that have "sticky" soles to provide traction—there are several websites where these can be ordered if you use the search term "dog booties." There are booties for sports, hiking, and snow, and most would be appropriate for an older dog inside. After all, you wouldn't let your grandmother go down slippery wooden stairs in socks—that's a recipe for a 911 call right there! If your dog must go "barefoot," however, remember to trim the fur between the pads on the bottom of her feet—fur flattened over the pads will prevent whatever traction her rough pads can provide. Another option to provide more traction and stability for your older dog is a great product called "Dr. Buzby's Toe Grips" (toegrips.com)—these are rubbery rings that you slip over each claw. Dogs' claws actually provide some of the traction for ambulation, but don't work as well on hard floors—these rings increase that traction and prevent slipping.

There is one balance problem that is unrelated to damage to the hearing apparatus—it is called *geriatric vestibular disease* and is usually a temporary but severe disturbance of the balance mechanisms in the inner ear that occurs most often in older dogs. It is unclear what causes it—inflammation is present but no infectious cause has been found, although very similar symptoms occur with inner ear infections, which are generally an extension of middle ear infections. Dogs displaying the sudden onset of symptoms that include being severely off-balance, falling to one side while trying to walk, tilting the head to one side persistently, and have repetitive side-to-side movements of both eyes (called *nystagmus*) should be evaluated for infection and be given appropriate medications if an infection is found. If no obvious infection is present, antinausea medications should be given as these dogs have the symptoms of motion sickness, due to the constant whirling sensation, but those that are unable to eat or drink need to be hospitalized briefly for intravenous fluids until the symptoms subside. The most severe symptoms usually last only a few days, and then the dogs slowly get back to their normal balance and appetite over the next two to four weeks. Sometimes the head tilt will persist, however, and some dogs (like mine) live long enough to get geriatric vestibular disease more than once—I considered that a badge of honor for my dog!

Overall, the loss of your dog's hearing may be more traumatic for you than for her. For her, it might simply be confusing. Humans rely so much on our hearing for our sense of community that the thought of the loss of that vital sense in our dog is very upsetting—that's an example of anthropomorphism and is less useful than caninomorphism in this situation. If you try to understand what the world sounds like to your dog, you can find ways to keep the lines of communication open—which will also make *you* feel better and less distant from your dog as these changes take place. She will still feel close to you—after all, she still has the use of her sense of smell to keep track of you, which, despite some age-related changes, will allow her to compensate for her age-related hearing and visual losses in many ways.

18

DIMINISHING RETURNS

First man: My dog's got no nose! Second man: How does he smell?
First man: Awful! —*Monty Python*

Since the sense of smell and the sense of taste are so closely related, a continuation of that joke might read: "How does he taste? Bland!" The medical term for the inability to smell is *anosmia* while the term for the inability to taste is *ageusia*. The complete lack of either of these senses in humans is actually very rare, but when either of those do occur, the most common cause is illness or injury. What is much more common, in both humans and dogs, are gradual changes in these senses which are related to aging—and, of course, there are terms for that: *presbyosmia* and *presbygeusia*. Age-related alterations in these senses can be related to both changes in the nerves that detect the stimuli and changes in the brain that processes that information.

For both species, the decline in the olfactory cells in the nose has a greater impact on the sense of taste than actual aging changes to the taste buds in the tongue since the taste buds really aren't as important as most of us think anyway. As you know, much of what we taste when we consume food or liquid is due to the aroma of that substance which goes from the back of the mouth, up through the throat, and into the back of the nose to stimulate the olfactory nerves. This is why a cold can interfere with how food tastes, and since most of us have had colds, we can relate to what it might be like for aging humans and dogs as they lose some of the sense of taste. Luckily, however, that type of impairment is temporary and resolves once the cold resolves—aging changes are (unfortunately) permanent, but (fortunately) slowly progressive over many years.

In humans, taste buds diminish as people get older, usually starting at forty to fifty years of age in women and at fifty to sixty years of age in men—although why this starts later for men is unknown. As the taste buds atrophy and die off, they are not replaced. For humans, the first tastes that seem diminished are "sweet" and "salty," later followed by "bitter" and "sour." This can lead older people to start adding more salt or sugar to their foods, which is not always a great idea for those with diabetes or high blood pressure—but these changes occur so gradually, most people are unaware they are occurring. For dogs, it is unclear which specific taste buds or taste sensations are lost with age—more work has been done on age-related changes to their sensory super-power, the sense of smell. Since that sense is so much more powerful in dogs than it is in humans, significant deterioration in the sense of smell may take longer to occur but will have a disproportionately greater impact on the sense of taste in dogs compared to humans.

As with many aspects of aging, changes to the senses of taste and smell are often a combination of cumulative insults to the sensory apparatus over a lifetime, and, in humans, there are several health, lifestyle, and environmental factors that have been linked to changes in the sense of taste, probably as it is related to the sense of smell. These are: nasal and sinus problems, dental disease, smoking, and head or facial injury. These are probably important risk factors for dogs as well—and is yet another reason to stop smoking and to make sure your dog has regular dental care!

There are also many known changes to the olfactory structures in humans that occur with aging—these include direct damage to the mucus-secreting cells lining the nose, a decrease in the production of enzymes that maintain the health of those cells, a reduction in the number of cells lining the nose, atrophy of the sensory receptors, changes in the chemicals that transfer nerve impulses, protein and pigment deposits in the nerves leading from the nose to the brain, and changes in the parts of the brain that receive that information. Many of these structural changes have been found to occur in aged dogs as well; one study looking at dogs ten and nineteen years old found that olfactory atrophy and degeneration started at age fourteen but was very prominent by age seventeen.[1] For humans, approximately 50 percent of people between sixty-five and eighty years old have a decreased sense of smell, and this goes up to 62–80 percent of those over eighty years old.

Impairment in the sense of smell is associated with a decrease in cognitive abilities and memory decline, and is considered to be an early warning sign of diseases such as Alzheimer's disease and Parkinson's disease, as all of these disorders are related to the processing of the sensory information that the brain receives. In fact, tests that detect decline in olfactory function have been found to be more sensitive in detecting decline in cognitive function than many of the standard question-and-answer-type cognitive tests commonly used in aging humans. Although the link between olfactory health and brain health has not been investigated in dogs, the degree of olfactory impairment may be a valid indicator of the integrity of the aging canine brain, as there are many similar age-related neurodegenerative changes in the two species.

In an earlier chapter, I recommended finding activities for your dog that could take advantage of the natural instincts he possesses as either a member of a certain breed or merely as a member of the canine species. These activities were meant to provide him with mental stimulation, physical exercise, a sense of purpose, and confidence as well as habits that he could rely on as life goes on and some of the senses that give him a connection to the world—and you—diminish. For many of those activities—whether they be organized sports like "Barn Hunt" or at-home games like "hide-and-seek"—your dog's inborn and amazing sense of smell is the reason for his success at them.

Since your dog's sense of smell may decrease later than the other senses, you can use his familiarity with these activities, and his confidence in his own abilities to do them well, to reassure him that he is still very good at something, and also that he is still very connected with you. As the senses of vision and hearing decrease, he may become more and more tentative moving around, and his sense of smell will be ever more important in helping him know where he is (and where you are). Continuing any activities that allow him to flex his nasal muscles, as it were, could make him feel mentally stronger and more self-assured. In addition, since changes in the sense of smell could be indicators of overall brain health, you might be able to use his ability to do those smell-related activities throughout his life to monitor your dog's brain health as he ages.

On the outside, a dog that loses interest in such an activity or gets distracted easily might appear disobedient or bored, and his human might get frustrated or disappointed in him, which could certainly create anxiety in the dog. On the inside, this dog might just be unable to discern the scents that make the game possible, because he has terrible periodontal disease interfering with the ability to use the olfactory apparatus to detect the odors, or possibly because his brain is starting to have trouble processing the information. An alert dog owner who notices these changes in the dog's ability to perform these games could then look for physical causes, if any, that could be corrected, such as periodontal disease, or could have the dog evaluated for cognitive dysfunction (the veterinary term for canine age-related dementia) to see if there are any interventional strategies that could be used to slow down that process.

In addition, it helps to remember that a dog who is not smelling well will not be tasting his food well—this could lead to a change in appetite, or at least in the gusto with which he eats. If one is aware of this, it's easy to counteract this by making the food smell stronger. Warm food releases the volatile odorants in the food rapidly and helps them disperse quickly—just adding warm water or warm low-sodium chicken broth to dry food will do that, as will heating canned food in the microwave for just a few seconds (only until it makes a little crackling noise, but isn't hot). Adding herbs (such as oregano or rosemary) to the food can help create a stronger, novel odor to the food—and so will a little grated Parmesan cheese. Salt or monosodium glutamate won't really help (and may be harmful)—these are flavor enhancers, not smell enhancers, and an older, presbyosmic dog may not be interested in eating a food in the first place unless it smells strongly. Lack of appetite is an important sign of illness in dogs of all ages that should trigger a trip to the veterinarian, while lack of enthusiasm while eating could be a sign of illness or could be a sign of age-related decreases in the senses of smell and taste. Seeing if these simple strategies to intensify the smell corrects the problem can be a good indicator of the source of the problem and will be useful information for the veterinarian that evaluates your dog.

There is another reason to pay attention to your dog's ability to smell—for humans, the lack of the ability to smell, and, therefore, taste, can lead to a sense of isolation and consequent depression, since many aspects of life that people find enjoyable are diminished—such as the smell and taste of freshly baked bread, or the various memories invoked by certain odors or tastes. Caninomorphically, we could theorize that dogs, who get more information about their world from their sense of smell than any of their other senses, could feel similarly isolated and even depressed as that sense declines. When their vision and hearing diminish, their sense of smell becomes of greater and greater importance in locating their people, maneuvering in an unfamiliar environment, tasting their food, and maintaining their connection to the world outside their bodies. As that crucial sense decreases with age, that connection can decrease as well—which is why humans have to work harder and harder as our dogs get older to stimulate that sense, decrease insults to it, compensate for changes to it, and find other ways we can connect.

And in what other ways can we connect? How about that one last sense—the sense of touch? Touch is the first sense newborn humans use to gain information about the foreign world in which they have suddenly entered—and it may be the last sense we can still use when we leave it. It appears, to me, to be the most long-lived and persistent sense there is, and doesn't seem to diminish with age as fast or as far as the other four. This isn't to say that there are not age-related changes to the sense of touch—there are—but these seem to be most pronounced in the set of receptors that process and define the *facts* (hot/cold, sharp/dull) of touch. Some of these changes occur because the skin's sensitivity decreases—this occurs for several reasons: the numbers of sensory receptors in the skin decrease with age, the skin becomes less taut, skin elasticity is lost, and, in addition, tissue and fat loss is just below the outer surface of the skin.

This means that older people, and dogs, have more trouble as they age in distinguishing differences in textures—for dogs, who have their second-highest number of sensory nerves in their feet, this means that older dogs may not be able to tell whether the surfaces they are walking on are rough or smooth, burning hot in the summer or slippery with ice in the winter, dangerous with broken glass or safely soft with grass. In addition to this decreased ability to discern textures, aged people, and dogs have a decreased sensitivity to pain, and may sustain an injury, such as a cut, without being aware of it—or showing the symptoms of it so that someone else will become aware of it. The high temperature of a heating pad, for example, may not cause enough discomfort to warn an older dog to move before his skin is burned. These cuts and burns can go undetected until they are infected or cause severe debility. Paradoxically, the decreased touch sensitivity that older humans and dogs experience lead to a delayed reaction to being touched by another person, and then, an exaggerated, startled reaction to it. This can give the other person the impression that the older person or dog does not want to be touched, so opportunities for elders to be connected to the world by touch might decrease—and that can lead to "touch hunger."

Ironically, however, this can occur just at the time that touch is most needed, and could be at its most therapeutic, since the most long-lived aspect of the sense of touch may be the pathway that deals with the social and emotional information about touch. This is the type of information that is processed in the areas of the brain devoted to pleasure and social bonding, which then trigger a release of endorphins and oxytocin, the so-called bonding hormone. I think those "caress fibers" live on as long as we do, no matter how little else we can feel, see, hear, touch, smell, or taste. Perhaps this is because we humans are, at base, social creatures, with the instinct to seek out and communicate, via any way we can, with others. Well, fortunately, so are our dogs. They have both a similar need and a similar ability to connect with us, and to know we are connected to them. Keep that line of communication open and busy throughout your dog's life, but use it more and more often as the other lines develop age-related static.

It is actually pretty easy—just pet your dog. But now that you know that, once he is older, he will have a decreased sensitivity to pressure and could have a delayed reaction to it, you will need to modify *how* you pet him. You may want to catch his eye before you touch him, so he won't be startled, or begin with a light touch, using the flat of your hand instead of the tips of your fingers, and gradually increase the pressure until he is aware of it. Use your flat palm to slowly touch all areas of your dog's body with long smooth strokes.

At the same time that you are using this massage to tell your dog something, you can use it to let your dog tell *you* something. Pay attention to what you are feeling, including all the layers, from the fur through the skin, fat and muscle, all the way down to the bone—if you have been doing this all through your dog's life during your monthly physical checks, you will have some idea of what has been normal for your dog's body throughout the years. Now, notice any differences in body surface warmth, in touch sensitivity, areas of swelling, parts where the muscles are more tense or smaller in bulk. Also, look and feel for changes in the thickness or quality of the fur, the texture of the skin, any lumps under the surface or bumps on the skin.

The production of oils for the skin decreases with age, causing scaly skin and dry fur, and the hair follicles can atrophy, leading to hair loss, but, although these are normal aging changes, there are also some illnesses that lead to changes in the skin and coat in older dogs—this is why changes in skin and fur should be brought to your veterinarian's attention, along with any new bumps you detect during your massages. A retrospective study showed that older dogs are more likely to have a diagnosis of tumors on or under the skin, with the ages of ten to fifteen years being the most common age range for these to appear.[2] Many of these are benign, but some are cancerous, and the only way to know the difference is for your vet to check them out. Keep using your physical exam notes to show to your veterinarian, and refer to your old ones to see what is really new and what is not.

Besides helping you see the early warning system for illness in your dog, massage can also help you calm him. Since many dogs have an increase in anxiety as they age, due in part to changes in their sensory abilities, massage is the perfect way to reinforce your connection at the same time that you decrease his stress. When you notice your dog is anxious, try using a stroke similar to petting in order to relax him. First, lightly rest your flat palm on the top of his head or neck, then make long, sweeping strokes along the length of the spine and all the way down the tail. Then, repeat this several times, stroking slowly but gradually increasing the pressure with each pass—although it is important not to press straight down on the lower part of the back, which can be painful if the back or legs have arthritis. Last, rest one hand on the base of your dog's head and the other on the pelvis (the slightly higher part of the back which is above his back legs). According to canine massage therapists, these two areas correspond to the parts of the spinal cord that control the rest and relaxation responses of the body. Remember that doing this may do you some good as well, since, while you are petting and massaging your dog, he is (sort of) petting you—the feel of your dog's fur and the warmth of his skin are simultaneously stimulating your C-fibers, too, and your own endorphins will increase. Dogs were, after all, invented way before Prozac!

19

STICKY WICKETS

I don't deserve this award, but I have arthritis and I don't deserve that either. —Jack Benny

It's a fact of life—our bodies and gravity aren't always the best of friends over time. Like many other things, the age-related changes in our joints that cause stiffness and pain are a consequence of cumulative insults over a lifetime—mainly to the cartilage inside each joint. Throughout our lives, every step we take, every landing after every jump we make, every fall we sustain has an impact—literally—on our joints and bones. If we carry extra weight, the force with which we hit the ground is greater—you can blame Sir Isaac Newton and his law of Universal Gravitation for that—and strength of the blows to our joints produced by every step, landing, and fall will increase in magnitude. Add to that any joint instability from poor formation of the joints, any defect in the formation of the cartilage within the joint or any previous ligamentous tear within a joint and the result will be greater wear and tear within the joints, and the ultimate outcome will be arthritis, or, more, specifically, *osteoarthritis* (OA). I suppose it would help to review what, actually, *is* a joint: joints are the areas where two or more bones meet. Most joints are mobile, allowing the bones to move. Joints consist of the following:

- *Cartilage*—this is a firm, rubbery material that covers the end of each bone at a joint. Cartilage provides a smooth, gliding surface for joint motion, helps reduce the friction of movement within a joint, acts as a cushion between the bones, and provides shock absorption.

- *Synovial membrane*—a tissue called the synovial membrane lines the joint and seals it into a joint capsule. The synovial membrane secretes synovial fluid (a clear, sticky fluid about the consistency of egg whites) around the joint to lubricate it.
- *Ligaments*—tough, elastic bands of connective tissue surround the joint to give support and limit the joint's movement.
- *Tendons*—tendons (another type of tough connective tissue) on each side of a joint attach muscles to bone and control the movement of the joint.
- *Bursas*—fluid-filled sacs, called bursas, between bones, ligaments, or other adjacent structures help cushion the friction in a joint.

"Arthritis" is often used as a general term to refer to any joint pain or stiffness—but there are actually over 100 forms of arthritis in humans (far fewer are recognized in dogs). In the United States, more than 50 million adults and 300,000 children have some type of arthritis, making arthritis the leading cause of disability in America. In dogs, it is estimated that 20 percent of the adult dog population is affected by arthritis in at least one joint.

Osteoarthritis is a joint disease that mostly affects cartilage—cartilage consists of specialized cells (*chondrocytes*) mixed with a fibrous protein (*collagen*) plus an elastic protein (*elastin*), held together by a supportive grid (*extracellular matrix* or ECM), which is, itself, produced by the chondrocytes. This cartilage matrix is composed of large protein molecules called *proteoglycans*, plus collagen, and is 80 percent water. Cartilage does not contain nerves or blood vessels, and nutrients to the chondrocytes are supplied only by diffusion, which is aided by a pumping action that occurs when the cartilage is compressed. Chondrocytes are bound to the underlying tissue, and can't migrate to areas of damage, so cartilage is not able to repair itself well, and tends to create scar tissue at sites of damage.

Inside the chondrocytes, there are enzymes and *cytokines* (small protein cells that provide communication between cells) which are, normally, inactive, but are produced in response to injury. When they are released, the cytokines stimulate the chondrocytes to release several different enzymes that degrade the collagen, elastin, and the matrix of the cartilage itself. These substances, along with other cytokines that increase inflammation, are pumped out of the cartilage into the fluid within the joint when it bears weight. When the cells that line the joint (*synoviocytes*) are exposed to these abnormal substances, they respond by producing their own inflammatory chemicals to combat them. Once the joint bears weight again, both groups of inflammatory substances are pumped back into the cartilage, where the chondrocytes react to the "foreign" chemicals produced by the synoviocytes, and then both go back out with the next weight-bearing event, and on to the next battle between the joint chemicals—and the inflammation cycles onward and upward. Why can't they all just get along?

It seems paradoxical that the processes that occur within the joint are more predisposed to inflammation and damage than repair. Actually, the inflammatory response is a natural defense mechanism that is triggered whenever body tissues are damaged in any way which prevents the spread of damaging agents to nearby tissues, disposes of cell debris and pathogens, and sets the stage for the repair process. With injury to cartilage, the chondrocytes can heal themselves to an extent, but they are regenerated very slowly, in part, due to their lack of a blood supply. Normally, within a joint, homeostasis (remember that term?) prevails and there is a balance between forces that damage the cartilage and forces that repair it. With aging, homeostasis loses out to catabolism, and damage wins out over repair. How does this happen?

- As the cartilage ages, there is decreased production of proteoglycans by the chondrocytes along with a loss of HA, GAGs, and water from the matrix.
- The cartilage, as a result, becomes less elastic with less ability to absorb shocks, and any minor trauma can produce cracks in the cartilage and chondrocyte damage.
- These surface cracks expose collagen fibers within the cartilage to wear and tear, and some cracks can extend into the deeper layers of the cartilage all the way to the underlying bone.
- Enzymes are released which further break down cartilage matrix and collagen.

- These enzymes and the products from cartilage breakdown initiate inflammation within the joint fluid that further increases
cartilage destruction and inhibits new matrix production.
- All of these changes contribute to decreased resiliency of the cartilage and increased hardness of the underlying bone.

Therefore, in osteoarthritis, the cartilage breaks down, causing pain,
swelling and problems moving the joint. As OA worsens over time,
bones may break down and develop growths called bone spurs (*oste-
ophytes*). Bits of bone or cartilage may chip off and move around in the
joint (known charmingly in the medical profession as "joint mice"). In
what is called "end-stage" osteoarthritis, the cartilage wears away and
bone rubs against bone, leading to joint damage and a *lot* of pain.
Interestingly, the pain that is felt with arthritis does not originate from
the damaged cartilage, since it has no sensory nerves, but comes from
the underlying bone.

This type of arthritis can happen in any joint, but, in humans, it
occurs most commonly in the hands, knees, hips and back. In dogs,
some of the most common joints affected are the metacarpal-phalan-
geal joints of the front feet (specifically, the second and the fourth
ones)—on your hands, these would be the big knuckles between the
bones of the palm and the bones of your forefinger and your ring finger.
This, by the way, is a good thing to remember when you are trimming
your older dog's nails—compressing those joints while holding the paw
for nail trims will cause pain. Other joints in dogs that are prone to
arthritis are the hips, shoulders, back, and knees. Risk factors for the
development of arthritis in humans as well as dogs include:

- increased weight
- increased age
- poor formation of the joint, as found with hip or elbow dysplasia
- previous joint injury that causes joint instability, such as anterior
cruciate ligament (ACL) rupture inside the knee
- genetic defects to joint cartilage that cause it to be fragile enough
to chip off—an example of this is *ostoechondritis dissecans* (a
cartilage defect in the shoulders more common in certain large
breed dogs)

- stresses on certain joints due to conformation, like "knocked knees" in people or the crooked joints that characterize certain breeds of dogs, such as Bassett Hounds
- stresses on certain joints from repetitive motions due to certain jobs or sports

Degenerative arthritis develops slowly over time and its symptoms can be insidious. Warning signs of osteoarthritis are:

- stiffness in a joint after being inactive for a long time, which decreases with activity
- stiffness or pain in a joint after overuse, or which increases after rest
- swelling or tenderness in one or more joints
- a crunching feeling, or crackling/grating sound, when a joint bends and straightens

In dogs, symptoms of arthritis can be subtle, and can require some extra vigilance to detect. For example, early in the development of arthritis, a dog may occasionally be reluctant or hesitant to perform some tasks or activities, such as jumping into the car or off the couch, going up or down a flight of stairs, or performing a well-rehearsed trick that requires standing up on the back legs or getting up from a sitting position. One might notice that a little extra "oomph" is required for a dog to arise from a prone position, and that he then takes a few stiff-looking steps until the joints "warm up" with activity and move normally. With arthritis in the bones of the neck, a dog might not bend her neck backward and upward enough to look up at her owner's face five feet above her, and might seem inattentive or uncaring. Bending the neck down to a food or water bowl on the ground may be difficult or painful, and the legs may have to be placed further apart to lower the body, and then slide due to the abnormal position. This can lead to decreased food or water consumption.

When a dog has "sticky" joints, more effort and strength is needed to move them, and the leg position may be angled differently, interfering with proprioception (the knowledge of where the limbs and body are in space), so some older dogs can just look clumsy rather than stiff. Arthritic dogs can be more prone to tripping because they are just a little too stiff or weak to raise their feet high enough to get over a small rise in the walking surface, like a threshold in a doorway or a tall clump of grass in the yard. A dog with hip arthritis may have trouble maintaining the crouched, hunched position that is required for defecation, and be unable to fully empty the rectum—this can lead to accidents in the house in a previously house-trained dog, especially since there is often an age-related decrease in sensation "down there." The same difficulty may be experienced with urination in the male dog that has to lift a leg that has a sore hip, or a female that needs to squat for a long time to empty the bladder. These dogs aren't having trouble remembering the house-training rules they learned so long ago or being deliberately disobedient—their bodies just may be not letting them comply with the rules anymore.

With arthritis, there is a vicious cycle that occurs: because there is inflammation and degradation within the joint, there is increased pain with movement, and movement (i.e., exercise) is avoided. This leads to decreased use of muscles, and the unused muscles get thinner and weaker. As muscles atrophy, the metabolic rate goes down, fewer calories are used so that the extra calories that are consumed are stored as fat, and the body weight increases. As the stiff, painful joints are required to move around a heavier body, they sustain greater concussive forces, sustain more damage, create more inflammation, and produce more pain—and the cycle continues. What's a dog owner to do?

DO DUE DILIGENCE

Continue to assess the risk factors for arthritis throughout your dog's life. Refer to the risk factor analysis you have made and refer to it often—is her breed prone to crooked joints, sliding kneecaps, poorly formed hips, knees or elbows, crooked legs, back problems, or cartilage defects? Ask your veterinarian to evaluate her, specifically, for those potential problems. If any are found, ask what you can do to minimize their effects, or even correct them while she is young, *before* cartilage damage occurs and the cycle of arthritis starts.

As life goes on, injuries to joints and the ligaments that hold them together can occur and unstable joints will have a greater risk of developing arthritis. An undiagnosed, and therefore, unrepaired ACL tear, for example, will lead to chronic joint instability and arthritis in that knee even in the younger years, whereas early diagnosis and repair can prevent it. Consult your veterinarian for appropriate early intervention for any joint injuries or congenital abnormalities, or any symptoms that you think might be due to arthritis, since other disorders, such as tick-borne illnesses, bone cancer, nerve problems, and back problems can have similar symptoms but very different treatments. Once the arthritis snowball starts rolling, however, it's hard to stop it, although you might slow it down. There is, unfortunately, no cure for arthritis, only control of the pain and degenerative changes that result. That doesn't sound so good, does it? So, do what you can to prevent it or delay its onset for as long as possible.

DON'T WAIT ON THE WEIGHT

Increased body weight is a significant risk factor for the development of arthritis—and a significant perpetuating factor once it develops. What's your dog's body condition score? What was it earlier?—this is when looking at the previous years' physical exam records that you have compiled will be helpful. Has your dog spent a significant part of her life being overweight? If so, her risk of age-related arthritis is greater. Is your dog overweight now? If so, no matter how old she is, take steps to reduce the amount of weight she carries on her joints to slow down the potential concussive damage. Don't forget that adipose tissue itself contains chemicals that promote inflammation which may help to perpetuate the inflammation within the joints as well as other parts of the body.

BALANCE ACTIVITY WITH ABILITY TO REDUCE DISABILITY

Active, physically fit dogs tend to have a better quality of life even when they have osteoarthritis when compared to inactive, unfit dogs with a similar degree of arthritis. So, keep your dog moving and motivated with activities that keep her muscles—and mind—toned, since the more muscle she has to begin with, the less she has to lose, in a way. However, be mindful of her risk factors in choosing her activities throughout life so as not to increase her joint damage over time. If any injuries have occurred that could have created an unstable joint, the type of activity you choose for her may have to change. Sustained running or jumping on an unstable knee will traumatize the joint, so choose an activity that doesn't require repetitive motion or thrust with the back legs, such as swimming or hide-and-seek. If your dog is developing arthritis, it doesn't mean she can't exercise at all—in fact, she now needs activity even more—you may just have to shorten your exercise sessions, and be very watchful for any signs of pain during exercise or stiffness afterward. If you notice any, decrease exercise until the soreness has resolved.

Beware of the "weekend warrior syndrome"—this happened to my own dog once, and I have never forgotten it! My husband and I had just rescued a fourteen-year-old Golden Retriever, Ryder, and were concerned about him because he seemed extremely depressed during his first few weeks in our home. We knew nothing about his previous life—that is, until one day when my husband and I took him to a park where we played tennis. As soon as we hit the first ball over the net, a laser-bright, happy light switched on in his eyes and, after waiting until the ball hit the net and dropped down onto the court, he rushed onto the court to grab it and bring it to me. We realized he had been trained to do this, and, after that, we played on for a long time, hitting the balls into the net just so he could joyfully retrieve them for us. Once the balls were so wet with saliva that they sprayed us when we hit them, we put Ryder in the car, went home and then tried to let him out of the car—only to find he couldn't walk at all! After I got over the initial panicky thought that he was paralyzed, my more logical medical brain kicked in and realized that he—and we—had just overdone it. Once Ryder had rest, some pain reliever/anti-inflammatory drugs, and a little time, he was just fine—although he was very uncomfortable in the meantime. Dogs are so motivated to do what they love to do, and what they know their owners love them to do, that they will ignore pain and do too much—until they can't. That's where their wiser human keepers come in handy—so be smarter than I was and protect your dog from herself!

Remember that exercise in a person, or dog, with arthritis is a double-edged sword—exercise of the right type and in the right amounts can be very beneficial for arthritic joints, but too much exercise, especially if it involves impact on hard surfaces, can be harmful—as it was for Ryder. If you had arthritis and you wanted to get the best advice possible for developing an appropriate exercise program, you would probably go to a physical therapist or certified personal trainer. For advice in developing a good exercise program for your dog, you may find the veterinary equivalent in your city by looking for a Certified Canine Rehabilitation Therapist, who can design a combination of therapies to be done at the rehab facility and at home. For instance, one of the dogs mentioned earlier in this book, Lucy, was helped tremendously by hydrotherapy (a swimming treadmill)—she was a classic example of the vicious cycle of arthritis—her very arthritic hips, shoulders, knees and back had kept her from moving around, and her muscles, before therapy, were very atrophied and weak. Hydrotherapy strengthened her muscles, made her joints more supple, and gave her mobility—and her life—back.

FEED THE FLUID

So, you now know the fact that cartilage is not very efficient at repairing itself as well as some of the reasons why it can become damaged as it ages—but did you know that there are some ways to help it get more efficient at repair and remain less damaged? Since chondrocytes can only get nutrients through diffusion through their matrix, and since, as the cartilage ages, there is less water content in the matrix, as well as decreased production of the proteoglycans by the chondrocytes, it seems logical that the cartilage should remain more elastic and more resilient if we can do something to maintain moisture within the matrix, to support the chondrocytes, and to replace the proteoglycans (hyaluronic acid and glycosaminoglycans). That is indeed a good idea—and there are supplements for that. You may have heard of them, seen them advertised or even found them in your dog's food—they are *glucosamine* and *chondroitin sulfate* supplements (also called "chondroprotective agents") and the name says exactly what they are supposed to do—protect the cartilage.

Most oral dietary supplements combine glucosamine with chondroitin sulfate; glucosamine is harvested from the shells of shellfish or is manufactured, and chondroitin is usually obtained from the cartilage of animals, like cows, pigs, or sharks, or is made in the laboratory. These substances are found in healthy cartilage and are a major component of cartilage; they help it retain water, and thus help cartilage remain soft enough to get its nutrients through diffusion during that pumping action described earlier. There is one injectable chondroprotective agent for dogs, which is more expensive than the oral supplements, but works differently, longer, and, some veterinarians say, better. It is a polysulfated glycosaminoglycan under the brand name Adequan which works to prevent cartilage breakdown by inhibiting the enzymes of cartilage degradation during inflammation.

These supplements have been used in horses, cats, dogs, and humans, and many studies on their efficacy have been performed over the years, with varying results. Some studies have focused on glucosamine, others on chondroitin, others on a combination of the two. According to the Mayo Clinic's assessment of these supplements for human use, good scientific evidence supports the use of glucosamine sulfate taken by mouth to treat knee osteoarthritis and possibly other joints, although there is less evidence to support other joints compared to knee osteoarthritis. For dogs, there aren't many controlled trials, and even fewer double blinded ones, and many of them are based on subjective measures of mobility and pain as assessed by human observers—obviously, in veterinary medicine, some of the difficulties in studying these products lie in the inability of dogs to report how their joints are feeling. A placebo effect can certainly be present in veterinary medicine—all of us want our dogs to feel better, and we may see what we want to see—but a dog that can't jump into the car before using glucosamine/chondroitin sulfate supplements who, after a month on them, *can* jump in the car is not responding to what she *wants* medications to do, only what she *can* do.

These supplements help many of my patients, and have helped many of my own dogs, so I recommend them, although they don't seem to work as well if they are given in the later stages of arthritis. Therefore, I recommend them early in life to protect the joint cartilage if a dog has significant risk factors for the development of arthritis, has a lifestyle that requires long distance running on hard surfaces, has misaligned or unstable joints, or is significantly overweight. I usually recommend that all large-breed dogs start them around the age of 8, and smaller dogs at ten, and for any dog of any age that is showing the subtle signs of early arthritis as described above. It is important to know that they will not become effective for about a month after starting them, and that, even if you can't tell that your dog is moving better after starting them, they may still be slowing the age-related damage to her joint cartilage and are, in my opinion, worth continuing. Discuss the use of these supplements with your own dog's veterinarian, to see if and when they are appropriate for your dog, and to see which form (oral or injectable) is best for her.

One note—many forms of these supplements are available over-the-counter for both humans and dogs under many brand and generic names—the only difference between the canine and human forms are the flavorings—most of us humans don't appreciate beef-flavoring in our pills. But, buyer beware! There is no FDA regulation for supplements, and someone can put dirt in a bottle and no one will know the difference between that and a legit supplement—unless someone analyzes it—which *Consumer Reports Magazine* has done a few times over the years. The testers have checked various brands and generic glucosamine/chondroitin sulfate supplements for both humans and dogs, and found that some of the products had tablets that contained far less of the glucosamine or chondroitin than the label claimed. At least for the veterinary products, I believe that you get what you pay for—well-known companies, that have a reputation to maintain, tend to invest in quality control and are more likely to have reliably potent products. However, there are so many brands available that it is best to ask your veterinarian for guidance on choosing a brand.

There are also some diets at pet stores that do contain glucosamine—but, in general, they don't provide a high enough dose to be effective. Prescription diets are available that provide an adequate dose, but these, being "prescription," are available only at veterinary clinics or by prescription elsewhere. Not all of these are appropriate for all dogs with arthritis, since there are other medical conditions that may require a certain diet, so, again, discuss whether a prescription diet for joint support is appropriate for your own dog.

PUT OUT THE FIRE

The strategies described previously are meant to lessen, if possible, the risk factors for the development of arthritis, and decrease the severity and progression of arthritis. However, the greatest risk factor for the development of arthritis is one you *don't* want to eliminate—a long life! Some degree of arthritis is nearly inevitable in dogs, and humans, if they live long enough. What should you do if or when arthritis develops in your own dog? Well, osteoarthritis is a condition that causes pain and inflammation, so the best strategy to combat the consequences of arthritis is to lessen both parts of the problem. There is a group of drugs called *nonsteroidal anti-inflammatory drugs* (NSAIDs)—these drugs relieve both the pain of arthritis, and the inflammation.

How do they work? When tissue is damaged, it releases chemicals called prostaglandins, which are like hormones. These prostaglandins cause the tissue to swell. They also amplify the electrical signal coming from the nerves and increase pain. NSAIDs work by blocking the effects of certain enzymes which help create prostaglandins. By blocking one or both of these enzymes, NSAIDs decrease the production of prostaglandins, and this translates into less swelling and less pain from the tissue damage.

The most familiar of these is, simply, aspirin. For humans, aspirin does a good job of relieving pain and inflammation, but does come with the risk of stomach irritation—in dogs, aspirin does *not* do a good job of relieving pain, and comes with a much, much greater risk of stomach irritation. So-called doggie aspirin is currently being sold in pet stores and creates problems for veterinarians like me because a lot of my clients forget to tell me they are using it—and, if I were to prescribe another NSAID or corticosteroids for a dog that is already on aspirin, or has been given it within the past two weeks, the combination of the two types of drugs will causes significant stomach inflammation, even to the point of ulceration.

Different types of NSAIDs should not be used in dogs within two weeks of each other, and NSAIDs and corticosteroids should also not be used within two weeks of each other as they will gang up on the stomach lining. And, by the way, *do not* be tempted to use any over-the-counter-human NSAIDs for your dog—most are very toxic to the canine liver and kidneys, and can also damage the stomach lining.

Acetaminophen (Tylenol) is a type of human NSAID which inhibits a different enzyme and can be used in some dogs that have medical problems, like kidney disease, that make them unable to take other NSAIDs—but it should only be used under medical supervision.

There is one other human NSAID that is used (by prescription only) for certain types of cancer—but all other human NSAIDs should be avoided. If your veterinarian does prescribe an NSAID, and your dog does not respond as well as you'd hoped, ask about trying another to see if it works better—just remember that there will need to be a two-week wash-out period between the two, and another type of pain reliever, which is not an NSAID, may be needed during that time to keep your dog comfortable.

All NSAIDs have potential side effects, and should not be used in dogs that have certain medical problems, such as liver disease, kidney disease, stomach ulceration or blood clotting problems. Blood work should be monitored periodically to be sure no problems are occurring, but the possibility of side effects should not deter you from considering the use of these drugs for your arthritic and painful older dog since the improvement in her quality of life, in terms of better mobility and decreased pain, could vastly outweigh the risks.

If your dog's pain is not relieved by NSAIDs alone, or you or your vet are concerned about using NSAIDs for your dog, there are pain relievers that can be used. These are generally safe to be combined with NSAIDs or corticosteroids and can even be layered together for very painful conditions. There is no reason for your dog to have pain if you and your vet can do something about it, and it is common for an older dog who has increasingly severe arthritis to require increasing medication as time goes on, so don't be shy about asking your vet about pain relievers to add to the joint supplements and NSAIDs if you think your dog's pain is not being relieved adequately. The medications to ask about are: tramadol (a synthetic codeine analog), gabapentin (Neurontin—used in humans for nerve pain and seizures), and amantadine (Symmetrel—used for Parkinson's disease in humans). Although these prescription drugs are used for different medical conditions in humans, they do relieve moderate to severe pain in dogs and should be a part of the pain-control arsenal that keeps your dog moving comfortably through old age.

There is another type of pain control to consider using for your arthritic dog—the above-mentioned Lucy had a great reduction in her arthritis pain with acupuncture. This, too, is a growing field in veterinary medicine, and should be considered as part of the pain-relief tool box every owner of an arthritic dog should dig into. How does acupuncture work? Well, it is far beyond me to really explain it in detail—it is, after all, a complicated type of medicine that has been developing for thousands of years, and requires years of study to practice—and I did not study it. I do, however, believe it works for many medical problems, especially pain.

The way it works is that the application of needles in certain regions of the body stimulates the body's own healing processes, its own anti-inflammatory chemicals and its own pain relievers, while slowing the transmission of the sensation of pain from nerve to nerve. Many studies have been done on the use of acupuncture for a variety of human medical problems, and one study I thought was especially interesting showed that, for human cancer patients, acupuncture worked as well as, but no better than, conventional pain medications—however, this study also showed that, if acupuncture and conventional pain relievers were used together, they were better than either one used separately.[1] This study illustrates a key point—use whatever means you have at hand—supplements, NSAIDs, pain relievers, physical therapy, acupuncture, even chiropractic therapy, to keep your dog comfortable for as long as possible. These tools are all valuable individually in their own ways, but one shouldn't be used at the exclusion of all the others—and should really be used together, since the whole, in terms of quality of life for your arthritic dog, is much greater than the sum of its pain-relieving parts.

ONE FISH, TWO FISH, OMEGA-3 FISH?

There is one more, very simple, thing that may help prevent or lessen osteoarthritis in your dog—fish oils! Oils from cold-water fish, such as mackerel, salmon, herring, tuna, halibut, and cod, are a great source of *Omega-3 essential fatty acids*. The human (and canine) body is capable of producing all the fatty acids it needs—except for two: alpha-linolenic acid (ALA), an Omega-3 fatty acid, and linoleic acid (LA), an Omega-6 fatty acid. There are three main types of Omega-3 fatty acids:

- Eicosapentaenoic acid (EPA) and docosahexaenoic acid (DHA) come mainly from fish, such as salmon, mackerel, and tuna, so they are sometimes called "marine" Omega-3s.

- Alpha-linolenic acid (ALA), which is the most common omega-3 fatty acid in most Western diets, is found in vegetable oils and nuts (especially walnuts), flax seeds and flaxseed oil, leafy vegetables, and some animal fat, especially in grass-fed animals. It is important to note that, although humans absorb Omega-3 fatty acids from flax seed, dogs do not absorb them well from that source. ALA is generally used for energy, and conversion into EPA and DHA is very limited.

Since the body cannot make these fatty acids from scratch, they must be obtained from food, or if foods can't supply enough, from supplements. Nutritionists call Omega-3 and Omega-6 fatty acids "essential" fats since the body needs them for many functions, from building healthy cells to maintaining brain and nerve function. They are an integral part of cell membranes throughout the body and affect the function of the cell receptors in these membranes. They provide the starting point for hormones that regulate blood clotting, contraction and relaxation of artery walls, and inflammation, plus they bind to receptors in cells that regulate genetic function. Both types of fatty acids are "essential" for body function, but both compete for the same enzyme in order to work—and it seems to be important for the Omega-3 fatty acids to win this battle. Omega-3s are particularly beneficial as they block inflammatory chemicals (prostaglandins and cytokines) and also are converted to other anti-inflammatory chemicals (*resolvins*).

The current nutritional recommendation is to increase the consumption of Omega-3 enriched foods, by, for example, eating fatty fish twice weekly. It can be difficult, however, to obtain enough Omega-3s from diet alone—that's where supplements, like fish oil capsules, come in handy. For dogs in the United States and elsewhere, the amount of Omega-6 fatty acids supplied by most commercial diets is higher than the amount of Omega-3s, except for certain prescription diets meant to promote joint or skin health. So, for most dogs, supplements are "essential" in order to supply enough Omega-3s—this is important to know because the benefits of Omega-3 fatty acid supplementation for canine osteoarthritis, in addition to other health problems, are clear.

Several studies on dogs with osteoarthritis have shown an improvement in many of the signs of arthritis, either as measured objectively by the veterinarian researchers, or observed subjectively by their owners.

One showed improvement in the degree of lameness and increases in the amount of weight-bearing in the affected limb(s) by the end of the ninety-day test period after starting a food supplemented with Omega-3s.[2] Another study showed that the dogs in the supplemented groups significantly decreased their overall need for NSAIDs by the end of the test period, and, in another, most of the owners correctly guessed which group (the fish oil group or the placebo group) that their own arthritic dogs were in.[3] They reported that their dogs moved around better at home, and that their hair and coat had even improved—another great benefit of fish oils! A fourth study lasted for six months, and, according to the owners of the dogs fed the supplemented food, their dogs had a significantly improved ability to rise from a resting position and engaged in increased play activity by six weeks after the start of the supplementation, with improved ability to walk at twelve and twenty-four weeks, compared with control dogs.[4] Many studies in human arthritis have indicated similar benefits—a 2010 meta-analysis (a statistical technique for combining the findings from several independent studies) found that Omega-3 fatty acids significantly decreased joint tenderness and stiffness in patients with rheumatoid arthritis and reduced or eliminated NSAID use. Preliminary studies indicate it may have a similar effect on osteoarthritis. It is, as mentioned elsewhere, difficult to objectively assess improvement in certain medical conditions in dogs, since canine patients can't report changes in their symptoms like human patients can. However, studies such as these seem to point to an improvement in the signs and symptoms of osteoarthritis in dogs when supplementation with Omega-3 fatty acids is provided. There are, as will be discussed later, many other potential health benefits from their use.

So, how do you get them in your dog? Many preparations are available for veterinary and human use, either in capsule or liquid form. The liquid form is the easiest to give to dogs, since it can be mixed with the food and most dogs like the taste. The capsules made for people can be given to dogs as well, depending on the dose needed, although the capsules themselves are large, and may be difficult for smaller dogs to swallow. It can be a bit tricky to figure out how much fish oil to give—since most preparations contain a combination of Omega-3s and other fatty acids, including Omega-6s, in varying proportions, all of them will be added together to be given as a total on the label—most capsules for human use contain a total of 1,200 mg of fish oil, and those made for dogs vary in the total amount of fish oils they contain.

The key in figuring out a dose for your dog is to determine what proportion of that total is the Omega-3 component. This will be listed on the label as "EPA" and "DHA" and will be shown in milligrams. The two amounts together will be the total amount of Omega-3s that are contained in the capsule and this varies between brands—some capsules contain less than 200 mg of Omega-3s per 1,200 mg fish oil capsule, some contain 800 mg. I generally recommend that dogs receive approximately 10–20 mg per pound per day *of the Omega-3 component*, so my clients have to read a few labels and do a little math when they are in the stores choosing a product. The fish oil capsules and liquids made for dogs may be available at your veterinarian's office, and, if not, may be found online—again, these can vary in the concentration of Omega-3s, so look at the ingredient part of the label to figure out your dog's dose, not necessarily at the dose recommendation given by the manufacturer.

SCRUB IN

If your dog has any underlying conditions that could increase her chances of eventually having severe arthritis, intervene early in life, if possible—we have discussed many preventative measures already, but one we have not discussed is surgery. There are many structural causes of arthritis, other than aging, and some structural causes can be eliminated before arthritis occurs, while others can be improved, in order to lessen the severity of the arthritis that eventually occurs. I have already mentioned some procedures that can be done early in life to improve hip conformation and to stabilize kneecaps—other procedures can be done as well. These should, ideally, be performed as soon as possible to minimize the progression of arthritis, but can be considered even in middle to older age. These procedures fall into three general categories:

- removal of anatomic defects, such as bone fragments in the elbows (from bones that did not fuse properly during development) or joint mice (from bits of cartilage that have chipped off inside the shoulder joint)

- reconstructive procedures to eliminate joint instability and correct anatomic defects
- fusing of a joint (arthrodesis) to stabilize it in order to decrease pain (done most commonly in the "wrist" (carpus) of the front leg, but also in other joints

Surgery to correct or improve arthritic conditions in humans is done so commonly that we don't even think twice about it—and surgery should also be considered an option for arthritic dogs. For Americans, hip and knee replacements (also called *arthroplasty*) are among the most frequently performed operations in the United States—about one million of these are done each year, and a study done in 2014 by the Mayo Clinic showed that, as of 2010, an estimated 4.7 million Americans had undergone total knee replacement and 2.5 million had undergone total hip replacement. Although knee replacements for dogs are not currently an option, total hip replacements are frequently done on dogs with severe hip arthritis due to dysplasia. Most often, only one hip is replaced, but having even one hind leg upon which to comfortably bear weight, in addition to the two front legs, can significantly lessen the pain, improve the mobility, and, therefore, change the life of a dog with hip dysplasia.

For smaller dogs with severe hip arthritis, or for dogs in whom total hip replacement is not an option (due to finances or lack of qualified surgeons), the femoral head (the "ball" the ball-and-socket hip joint) can be removed—this may sound drastic, but is an option worth considering since, if you think about it, the joint can't hurt if it is no longer there. Since, as you now know, the pain of arthritis comes not from the damaged cartilage, but from the underlying bone, taking out the part of the joint that is grinding against the other part of the joint will eliminate the pain. Eventually scar tissue provides enough support to the thigh bone to mimic the support of the hip joint, and I have seen dogs that have undergone this procedure become so much more mobile, and happy, than they had been when they were living with a severely painful hip.

I always encourage my clients, and you, to explore all options available to improve the quality of life for an aging dog—lack of mobility, and pain, are life-limiting problems for many older dogs, particularly the large ones that can't be picked up to go outside. Lack of mobility is at the root of many of the health problems associated with advancing age—for humans and for dogs—and sometimes starts the "downward slide" into degeneration. Here's one more way to keep from going down that slide.

STEM THE TIDE

What is the opposite of degeneration? Regeneration! In both human and veterinary medicine, there is growing interest in the field of *regenerative medicine*. Regenerative therapy is aimed at encouraging the body's own reparative powers to heal an injury, regenerate tissue, combat ongoing damage and restore function. Regenerative medicine itself isn't new—bone marrow and solid-organ transplants are examples of this type of medicine, and the first ones were done decades ago. There are three aspects of regenerative medicine:

- *Rejuvenation*—boosting the body's natural ability to heal itself
- *Replacement*—using healthy cells, tissues or organs from a living or deceased donor to replace damaged ones
- *Regeneration*—delivering specific types of cells or cell products to diseased tissues or organs, where they will ultimately restore tissue and organ function

Earlier in this book, in the section that discussed how and why aging occurs, you read about stem cells and may remember that they are unspecialized cells that give rise to specialized cells. Stem cells are a key component of regenerative medicine since they have the ability to develop into so many different types of cells, such as skin cells, brain cells, and lung cells. You may also recall that stem cells within organs participate in tissue maintenance and repair after injury—but how do they do that? Stem cells are thought to repair tissues by:

- providing an anti-inflammatory effect
- being attracted to and migrating into damaged tissues
- recruiting other cells that are necessary for tissue growth
- assisting in the remodeling of tissue to decrease scar formation
- inhibiting programmed cell death (*apoptosis*)

- differentiating into a variety of tissues, such as bone, cartilage, tendons, and ligaments

Regenerative medicine uses stem cells from a variety of sources to regenerate and repair many types of tissue damage. Most commonly, the stem cells are isolated from a patient's own bone marrow or fat stores and then injected directly into the tissue that needs them—these types of stem cells (mesenchymal stem cells) are the ones most heavily researched and are utilized in both human and veterinary medicine. Regenerative medicine researchers are also studying other types of stem cells, such as embryonic stem cells, progenitor cells (such as those found in umbilical cord blood) and bioengineered cells (called induced pluripotent stem cells). In some research, a patient's own cells, from the skin, for example, are removed, then reprogrammed to give them certain characteristics, and then re-injected back into the patient to treat a specific disease.

This may surprise you, but stem cells have been used in veterinary medicine for many years, and, in fact, stem cell treatments are more available to pets than to people. Although research on stem cell therapy for human medical conditions is ever increasing, the U.S. Food and Drug Administration (FDA) has only approved the products for humans used in treatment of leukemia and other cancers that are related to blood-forming stem cells. By comparison, animal treatment involving stem cells is less regulated and has, therefore, expanded rapidly in the past ten years. Part of the reason for this is because the FDA does not require approval for therapies that are not drugs, and stem cells are not drugs, but substances that are taken from a body and injected, except experimentally, into the same body. The FDA is, however, starting (rightly so) to impose guidelines on the companies that process the stem cells, and this includes the performance of FDA-approved clinical trials as well as the adherence to certain procedures for safety and efficacy.

Originally, stem cells were mainly used to treat horses and dogs with injuries to, or defects in, their bones, cartilage, ligaments and tendons. The most common use has been for treatment of osteoarthritis, but research in the field is ongoing, and stem cells are being investigated for treatment of inflammatory bowel disease, chronic dry eyes (keratoconjuctivitis sicca) and autoimmune diseases. For dogs, the most common tissue from which the stem cells are extracted is adipose (fat) tissue, since it is so readily available. In most cases, the patient's own stem cells are injected back into the patient, but sometimes the adipose-derived stem cells are donated to another patient. Bone marrow has also been used as a source of stem cells for dogs, and so is umbilical cord blood, which is collected, for use by other dogs, after dogs have undergone C-sections.

In dogs, the most common condition treated with regenerative therapy remains osteoarthritis, and the ideal candidate for stem cell treatment is a dog in otherwise good health that suffers from arthritis but hasn't responded adequately to medications and supplements. The first step in stem cell treatment is the collection of fat cells from the dog's body—this is done under general anesthesia via a small incision through the skin behind one of the shoulders, where there is usually a fat pad, or into the abdomen, where there is ample fat to collect. After that, the fat is either shipped to a company in California (VetStem Biopharma) for extraction and concentration of the stem cells, or it is processed in the veterinarian's clinic, if that facility has a stem cell extraction unit (Medi-Vet Biologics). Once the stem cells are collected, they are injected into the affected joint or joints of the dog, with use of sedation and local anesthetics. A portion of the stem cells is often stored for future use, and some of these cells can be used to create new stem cells if the stored sample is being used up—this is helpful so that the dog does not have to go through the fat collection procedure again in order to have another treatment in the future. If effective, the treatment can be done again if the owners notice a reoccurrence of symptoms, which may happen one to three years after the therapy.

How effective is this? Not many good, sound scientific studies have been done so far, unfortunately, although several are currently underway. One good study was done in 2007 on dogs with hip arthritis—one group got stem cells injected into the hips, and the other group got saline injections.[5] Veterinarians and owners evaluated the dogs over time, and the veterinarians noted improvement of several symptoms in the group that received the stem cells, although they did not know which group received them. Interestingly, the owners of the dog didn't notice significant improvement. Another, more recent study showed objectively-measured improvement in the symptoms of hip arthritis after injection of stem cells, although this study showed the effects to diminish over a few months.[6] That being said, I believe that stem cells can work for many patients with arthritis—and this is because I saw stem cells bring amazing improvement in my own arthritic dog, Shrek. Whereas I realize that the placebo effect could color my judgment of the success of this therapy for my dog, I don't think my imagination created all the changes I saw in his activity level, amount of play activity, strength, exercise tolerance, and the absolute *joie de vivre* he displayed after the treatment.

Here's Shrek's story: In 2005, my husband and I adopted two Golden Retriever puppies (siblings) from the same Golden Retriever rescue group that allowed us to adopt Ryder, who had just passed away from cancer. We took them home at seven weeks of age, and, by eight weeks of age, I knew Shrek had problems—he would sit or lie down unless his princess-perfect sister, Fiona, was playing with him. It quickly became apparent that he not only had hip dysplasia but also had growth abnormalities of the bones in his front legs, causing them to become crooked. He underwent corrective surgeries on his pelvis and front legs at the age of seventeen weeks, which, thankfully, prevented his elbows and hips from eventually becoming dislocated. Despite surgical procedures, weight control, and supplements, Shrek still developed arthritis, although these interventions lessened its severity. In figure 19.1, you will see four hip X-rays: *Image A* shows normal canine hips—this happens to be Fiona at the age of one year—showing the "ball" of the joint to be well within the "socket." *Image B* shows Shrek's hips at the same age— you should see that the hip on the right of the image doesn't fit very deeply into the socket, because the socket is too shallow. *Image C* shows that, over time, the hip got partially dislocated because of the poor fit, became even more unstable, and the excessive motion damaged the cartilage. *Image D* shows what happens after a few years of joint instability—lots and lots of bone spurs which caused restricted motion in the joint and, sadly, much pain.

When Shrek was only two years old, he was no longer responding to NSAIDs or other pain medications, was no longer playing with Fiona or going up the stairs—so we tried stem cells, with the encouragement and support of the staff at our progressive clinic. I must admit, I was not very hopeful and was very, very skeptical—until I saw the change in him. About thirty days after the injections of the stem cells into his hips, knees, shoulders and bloodstream, I was in our backyard with the dogs

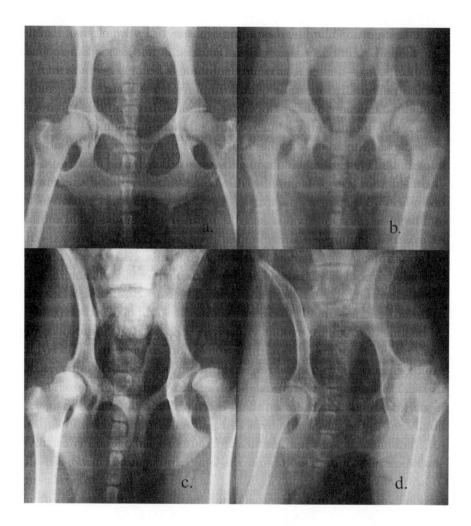

Figure 19.1.   Progression of Hip Dysplasia to Arthritis: (A) Normal hips (Fiona age 1); (B) Poorly formed hip on right side of photo (Shrek age 1); (C) Partially dislocated hip on right due to shallow socket (Shrek age 2); (D) Severe arthritis due to joint instability (Shrek age 8). Photos by author.

when my husband came home from work, parked the car in the detached garage, and came up to the backyard fence to say hello as he always did—and, much to our surprise, Shrek spontaneously stood up on his back legs and put his front paws on the top of the fence to say hello back! This was a dog that had *never* in his life jumped up on anything or anybody—his sister, Fiona, in contrast, had no problems in that regard! At sixty days after the treatment, I decided to test him and opened the hatch on my small car—and he jumped right on in! At ninety days, I gathered the staff at our clinic in the parking area, and opened the back door of our very tall SUV—and, again, he sailed in, to the applause of the crowd. My husband and I were astonished and very happy to see the improvement—but we were a bit unprepared for the sudden arrival of a dog who started to counter-surf and steal, not food, but anything that even remotely resembled a tennis ball. He suddenly became ball-crazy—as every good Golden Retriever should be—and wanted to play *all* the time. He still limped, due to his crooked legs, and was not as fast as his perfect sister, but he had become playful, energetic, and truly joyful. I don't think the placebo effect did all that—but I'm not sure *what* made him ball-crazy.

Shrek's story is certainly not as good as a scientific study, but it does illustrate a good point about novel therapies, such as stem cells, for osteoarthritis—if you feel that your dog's quality of life is being damaged by arthritis, or any other medical problem, it is within your power to change that. Don't just give up or remain satisfied with traditional therapies. The world of veterinary medicine is changing rapidly, and the therapies I describe now may eventually be eclipsed by new therapies that are only a glimmer in the eye of some researcher now—so, as time goes on, think outside the limits of current therapies and keep your mind open to new ones as your dog ages. You are, after all, your dog's health care advocate and life coach; remember, this might be the longest-term job you'll ever have, and you do have to keep up your skills!

20

FUZZY LOGIC

There are three signs of old age. The first is your loss of memory. I forget the other two. —Unknown

What is it that people fear the most about getting older? According to a survey done in the United Kingdom in 2014, the top five fears about aging are:

1. health issues
2. serious illness
3. a failing mind
4. becoming forgetful
5. losing independence

I find it interesting that two of those top five relate to the same thing—brain function. The pervasiveness of this particular fear was supported by a Harris Poll conducted online in 2014 which found that, of the two thousand respondents, an average of 73.5 percent of adults of all generations worry about what will happen to their memory as they age, and that 45 percent of all adults admit they are actually scared of aging. Not surprisingly, there is a medical term for the fear of aging: *gerascophobia*. Fortunately for most people, their worries about aging rarely reach the anxiety levels of a phobia, but do tend to become more severe right around that milestone birthday—the big five-o! As far as I know, no studies have been done on dog owners to assess their fears, if any, about the aging process in their dogs, but I suspect the results of such a study would show that the fears of dog owners would mirror their own fears about aging, with concerns about their dog's mental function being prominent among them. After all, our relationship with our dogs is dependent on our mutual ability to connect, to "click" when we look into each other's eyes, to respond to each other's cues, to perform all those same little rituals that make our bond different than everyone else's—and, if one of those two great minds can't think alike, the relationship shifts a little. Who wants that? Nobody—certainly not you, and, as much as I'd like to say your dog doesn't want that either, he probably isn't worrying about it at all—lucky him! But since you and I are, let's think of some ways we can help your dog hang on to as much of his mental juice as he can.

First, let's see what it is so many of us are afraid of—for most of us, it's *dementia*. Dementia is a general term that describes a set of symptoms that relate to impairment of *cognition*, which is a term referring to the mental processes involved in the acquisition of knowledge and comprehension. These processes include thinking, knowing, remembering, judging, problem-solving, language, imagination, perception, and planning. Dementia occurs when the brain is damaged by a disease such as Alzheimer's disease (AD) or by a series of strokes. The specific symptoms that someone with dementia experiences are dependent upon the parts of the brain that are damaged and upon the particular disease that is causing the damage. Those with dementia often have difficulties with some of the following:

- *Day-to-day memory*—trouble recalling events that happened recently
- *Concentrating, planning, or organizing*—difficulties making decisions, solving problems, or carrying out a sequence of tasks, such as cooking a meal (this is known as *executive function*)
- *Language*—inability to follow a conversation or find the right word for something
- *Visuospatial skills*—problems judging distances (such as on the stairs) and seeing objects in three dimensions
- *Orientation*—becoming confused about where they are or losing track of the day or date

In addition to these cognitive symptoms, people with dementia will often have changes in their mood, becoming frustrated or irritable, withdrawn, anxious, easily upset or unusually sad. AD is the most severe form of dementia, and, unfortunately, the most common. The cause has not yet been fully identified, but patients with AD have specific structural changes in their brains—they have *amyloid* plaques (an accumulation of an abnormal protein) between nerve cells (neurons) in their brain. Amyloid is a general term for protein fragments that the body produces normally. *Beta amyloid* (Aβ) is a protein fragment snipped from an *amyloid precursor protein* (APP). In a healthy brain, these protein fragments are broken down and eliminated. In AD, the fragments accumulate to form hard, insoluble plaques within brain tissue; amyloid also develops in the walls of blood vessels bringing oxygen and other nutrients to the nerve cells. These blood vessel abnormalities appear to lead to very small hemorrhages in the brain—this occurs to a certain extent in all aging brains, but, in dementia, including the dementia seen in AD, there are more areas of bleeding.

People with AD also have another structural problem in their brains—their brains contain *neurofibrillary tangles*, which are twisted fibers found inside the brain's cells. These tangles consist primarily of a protein called *tau*, which forms part of a structure called a *microtubule*. Microtubules help transport nutrients and other important substances from one part of the nerve cell to another and help nerve cells communicate. In AD, however, the tau protein is abnormal and the microtubules collapse. Together, the formation of amyloid plaques and neurofibrillary tangles are thought to contribute to the degradation of the nerve cells in the brain and the subsequent symptoms of AD. Much Alzheimer's research is aimed at figuring out whether one or the other of these two abnormalities is the major contributor to the dementia seen in AD, or if both are required. This is important for many reasons—especially for the development of drugs that could prevent, slow, or cure AD in susceptible individuals.

Aging dogs show many of the same cognitive changes as their aging human counterparts, including declines in learning, memory, visuospatial skills, executive function, and orientation. They also have many of the same degenerative changes to their brains and neurons. Just like in other parts of the body, degenerative changes in the neurons build up over time, because of mitochondrial dysfunction and oxidative damage.

Aging dogs have also been found to progressively accumulate beta-amyloid to form diffuse plaques outside their neurons as well as within the blood vessels of their brains. The amyloid plaques appear to be very similar to those of humans with AD, and, although dogs appear to have some tau abnormalities, they don't seem to develop fully formed neurofibrillary tangles.

Several key features of canine brain aging are very similar to that of humans—this has made the canine species an intense focus of research for use in the study of human brain aging, particularly because pet dogs share an environment and diet similar to their humans, and absorb many nutrients and medications in a comparable fashion. All of us will benefit from this research, particularly in the areas of prevention and therapeutics—but those of us who live with aging dogs get to benefit *twice* from the knowledge gained in this research since extrapolations from research on dementia in both species can potentially be applied in both directions.

You will be happy to know that cognitive decline in humans and dogs is *not* an inevitable consequence of aging, and much research has focused on which humans and dogs develop cognitive dysfunction and which do not. In terms of age-related cognitive function, aging humans and dogs appear to fall into three basic groups—those that do not show cognitive decline (these are known as "super-agers"), those that show moderate impairment in the completion of tasks that measure memory and learning, and those that are severely impaired and fail to complete any of those tasks. What makes the difference? Of course, that's what everyone wants to know—even those of us who are not gerascophobic! Risk factors for the development of dementia in humans include:

- genetics
- diabetes
- heart disease
- smoking
- depression
- chronic stress
- obesity
- physical inactivity
- mental inactivity
- periodontal disease

It appears that dogs share many of these risk factors, although no genetic predisposition to dementia has yet been found in dogs. What about smoking, you say? Well, of course, dogs don't smoke—but their owners do! Although a link between secondhand smoke and dementia in dogs has not been examined, the possibility of one should serve as another reminder to make sure people don't smoke around your dog (and you). Structurally, what changes in the brain as humans and dogs age and how might those changes relate to cognitive function? Some of these changes include:

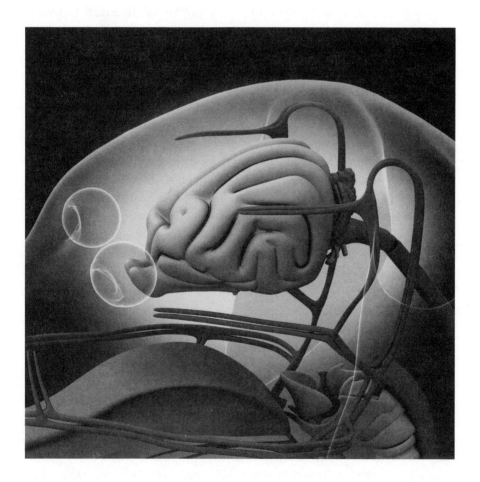

Figure 20.1.   The Canine Brain. Thinkstockphotos.com/*decade31*.

- Atrophy of the *cortex*—this is wrinkled surface of the brain and is a specialized outer layer of the *cerebrum* (see figure 20.1). Certain areas are strongly linked to certain functions, including the interpretation of sensations (sight, sound, smell, taste, and touch), the generation of thought, the ability to solve problems and make plans, the formation and storage of memories, and the control of voluntary movement.
- Widening of the *ventricles*—these are spaces between brain tissue that are filled with cerebrospinal fluid.
- A decrease in the overall volume of *white matter* and *gray matter*—white matter is called that because of the pale color of this fatty insulation-like coating around the long stalks of neurons, which increases the speed of transmission of electrical impulses through them. Grey matter, which is composed of the nerve cell bodies (where the cell nuclei are located) isn't coated with myelin—the brain's white matter can be thought of as a set of telephone wires which enable communication between the gray matter "thinking regions."
- Areas of increased density, as shown on MRI, within the white matter of the brain that indicate changes in the coating (myelin) around nerves as well as blood vessel damage.
- Degenerative changes to the nerve cells—due to the accumulation of toxic proteins, including beta amyloid, or damage to components of the neurons, such as the lipids, proteins, or DNA, because of the accumulation of free radicals. Younger brains appear to be able to provide enough antioxidant activity to keep pace with this accumulation, but older brains appear to be unable to keep up.
- Reduced rate of replacement of aging neurons with new ones—as cells within nerves die off naturally (apoptosis), they are replaced, albeit slowly, in younger brains. This is called *neurogenesis*, and the rate of replacement gets progressively slower with age.

Cortical atrophy has been shown to be associated with changes in cognition in both humans and dogs, with those showing the greatest amount of atrophy performing more poorly in tests of learning and memory. In dogs, MRI studies suggest that certain brain areas are especially prone to changes—the *prefrontal cortex* loses tissue volume at an earlier age (at approximately eight to eleven years of age) than does the *hippocampus* (after eleven years). The hippocampus plays an important role in the consolidation of information from short-term memory to long-term memory and in spatial navigation; it is also part of the limbic system, which is involved in emotion. In AD, the hippocampus is one of the first regions of the brain to suffer damage, making memory loss and disorientation among the early symptoms. Atrophy is found to some extent in the neurons of all aging humans and dogs but is most pronounced in the brains of patients with AD.

In dogs, the numbers of nerve cells in the hippocampus of young dogs (three to four years of age) were compared to the numbers found in the same region of older dogs (thirteen to fifteen years of age) and it was found that the old dogs had about 30 percent fewer neurons in one area. It was found that the number of neurons was correlated with cognitive function—dogs with higher numbers of hippocampal neurons performed a visual discrimination task with fewer errors. Another study found that older dogs have a drastically reduced rate of replacement of the neurons that have died off and that the degree of neurogenesis was associated with cognitive function—the dogs with fewer new neurons had higher error scores in measurements of learning and memory, as well as poorer learning ability.[1]

Researchers have developed many tests to detect changes in the thinking ability of dogs, and have been able to relate those changes to specific areas of the brain that have changed structurally over time, in order to predict what cognitive changes dogs might be expected to have at certain ages. Some of these tests will seem a little convoluted, but are designed to be done in a controlled, laboratory setting in order to produce results which can be reproduced and validated. You won't be doing these types of tests on your dog, but you may relate behavioral changes you are observing in your aging dog to the findings of this research, especially if you have been, as I hope, playing games with your dog throughout his life that involve thinking, memory, and planning. These activities will not only have provided your dog with physical and mental exercise (which could potentially help him be a "super-ager") but can now provide you with ways to assess his cognitive abilities as he ages. If you do detect changes, you may use this knowledge to modify some of your activities to compensate for changes in his memory or learning abilities. This will help keep him stimulated and can prevent the frustration that might result (in both of you) if some of the old games can't be done as well anymore.

In general, two categories of tests have been devised to assess cognitive function in aging dogs—one measures the ability to acquire new information and then use it (i.e., learning), while the other measures memory—the length of time that the new information is retained and used. Memory formation itself has three phases—an initial phase when the memory is acquired, an intermediate phase, and a consolidation/ storage phase which leads to the formation of long-term memory. Although learning and memory would seem to be two halves of the same coin, they aren't—learning and memory are considered separately, since a dog (or person) may have a good memory but be unable to learn quickly, or can acquire new skills quickly, but not retain them for long, since he has a poor memory. This is important because a gradual decline in memory and a decrease in the rate of learning occur with normal aging, but selective memory loss may signal the onset of dementia. Mild cognitive impairment—that is, problems in memory, language, thinking, and judgment that are greater than normal age-related changes—is thought, in humans, to signal the start of AD. As the disease progresses, an inability to take in new information, added to the loss of recall, worsens and these both interfere with the ability to solve problems and organize information.

Within these two categories, there are many tests that measure specific types of learning and memory in dogs. Tests that measure learning include:

- spatial learning (the ability to locate objects in space)
- egocentric spatial learning (dogs were rewarded for choosing the object closest to their own body)
- landmark learning or attention to the position of an object in space (dogs were rewarded for choosing the object, out of a choice of two, that was closest to another object—the "landmark")
- size concept learning (dogs were rewarded for always choosing either the larger or smaller object in a group of two identical objects so that they demonstrated that they learned the concept of "size")
- object recognition (dogs were presented with an object, then, after a few seconds, presented with the same object along with a

new one—they were rewarded if they chose the new object—this demonstrates the ability to classify objects)

- oddity discrimination learning (dogs were presented with three objects, two identical and one different—the dogs were rewarded for choosing the "odd" one—this shows the ability to pay attention to details like size, shape, color, and brightness)
- reversal learning (once a task was learned, the dogs were asked to learn to do it the opposite way, then assessed for their ability to make the change)

Tests that measure memory use those same tasks, but are modified to either increase the amount of information that the dogs must hold in working memory to do the task correctly, or increase the amount of time they must remember it to complete the test.

All of the tests of learning and memory listed earlier have been found to gradually become more difficult as dogs age, but it turns out that one of the most consistent cognitive deficits in aging dogs is the inability to acquire and use spatial information. This correlates well with the observation that the prefrontal cortex, which is involved with visuospatial working memory, begins to atrophy in dogs at eight to eleven years of age, although testing shows the impairment can start as early as six and seven years of age. However, the ability to learn simple tasks which involve visual discrimination is not impaired with age. Tasks that involve *procedural learning* are also done well by aging dogs—procedural learning refers to knowledge of skills that involve several steps, such as ringing a bell to indicate the need to be let outside. None of the learning and memory deficits appear to be related to age-related sensory or mobility changes.

Other studies have shown that impairment of executive function—the ability to plan and organize information—may be another early indicator of cognitive dysfunction in dogs and may precede any other obvious cognitive impairment. Executive function is controlled primarily by the frontal lobes of the brain. One of the features of executive function is *inhibitory control*—this is the ability to attend to a current task and to tune out distractions from the outside world (the surrounding environment) and from the "inside world" (previous memories or habits). Lack of inhibitory control is thought to lead to problems processing and understanding new information, and a subsequent inability to solve problems. Problems in "reversal learning tasks" indicate problems with executive function, as the dog may continue to exhibit the behavior that was previously rewarded even when a new one is being rewarded.

How does this relate to your dog? Well, many of the activities you enjoy with your dog—whether they are simple day to day routines, games, or formal sports—depend on your dog's ability to learn and remember where objects are in space, to learn and remember the location of objects in relation to his body or some other landmark, to recognize objects, to discriminate between different objects, to learn new tasks, to demonstrate skills that involve several steps, to solve problems, to organize information, and to tune out distractions. As you perform those activities with your dog throughout his life, you may start to notice changes—is your dog still a good learner, but can't remember things for long? Or is his ability to learn decreased, but his memory good? Is he, at the age of six to seven years of age, starting to forget where things are in your house? Or how to let you know when he needs to go outside, looking perhaps at the side of the door to the outside that doesn't open (the hinge side)? Does he remember the route you always take on walks, showing that he recognizes landmarks? Does he recognize his toys and what to do with them, or recognize when you have provided him with a new toy that he hasn't seen before? Does he recognize familiar people or dogs? Is he interested in, or indifferent to, new people or dogs? Can he learn a new trick quickly (old dogs really can learn new tricks) and remember how to do it the next day, or do you need to teach it again?

It is important at this point to remember—again—that not all dogs will develop full-blown dementia, also known as Cognitive Dysfunction Syndrome (CDS)—and, hopefully, with the help of the knowledge you have gained in this book, you will have managed your dog's risk factors for the development of CDS and other health problems so well that you won't have to worry about it anyway! But, just so you know—the overall incidence of CDS was found in one study to be 14.2 percent in dogs over the age of eight years. Breaking it down by age group, the distribution was: 5 percent in ten- to twelve-year-old dogs, 23.3 percent in twelve- to fourteen-year-old dogs, and 41 percent in dogs over fourteen. This was from an internet-based study that asked readers of *DogsLife* magazine to fill out a questionnaire designed to detect signs of CDS—

interestingly, only 1.9 percent of these dogs had been diagnosed by their veterinarians as having CDS. Veterinarians don't live with their patients and can't see all the day to day changes that occur—but *you* do, and, as this study shows, you can diagnose it much earlier than they can. CDS is rarely diagnosed by veterinarians before the age of eleven years, but the signs in some dogs may be seen by observant owners (like you!) much earlier. However, some signs of learning or memory problems that can be difficult to differentiate from other causes of behavior changes, such as age-related sensory changes, changes in mobility, and medical conditions. Many owners of older dogs don't discuss any behavior changes with their veterinarians since they (incorrectly) assume that these changes are the inevitable, and untreatable, consequences of aging.

Why is this important? As with many things, early detection and early intervention are crucial. If the behavior changes are due to a medical problem, the earlier that problem is addressed, the better the chances of curing or, at least, minimizing it. If the behavior changes are due to age-related sensory changes, or mobility problems, the environment can be modified to make it easier for the dog to move around, and supplements or medications can be started. This is one of the reasons that we spent so much time in this book learning about the five senses, about the health and behavior of your individual dog, and about how that changes with age. This knowledge helps you categorize the various changes you see in your aging dog and gives you the tools to deal with them. If there are changes you can't attribute to one of those other categories, you may be seeing early signs of cognitive impairment—and the earlier those signs are recognized, the earlier that interventions that could slow the progression of the problem—or even improve it.

First, however, let's go over the general behavioral changes that are seen in dogs with CDS. They include:

- spatial disorientation
- confusion
- altered learning and memory—common signs are house soiling or lack of response to previously learned commands
- changes in activity—either decreased or increased, and, when increased, dogs may show repetitive or purposeless activity, such as continually walking around the house

- changes in social relationships—demonstrated by being indifferent to owners, uninterested in new people or dogs, or being overly clingy
- altered sleep-wake cycles—such as night time waking
- increased anxiety
- restlessness
- decreased interest in eating
- irritability
- decreased perception of, or responsiveness to, stimuli

You can see that it could be difficult for most dog owners to tell whether, for example, a decrease in the perception of sound, or changes in appetite, are due to changes in the senses of hearing and taste, or are due to brain changes—but *you* aren't most dog owners! You have been given the tools to tell the difference—and are about to get some more.

At the end of this chapter, you will have a new exam form to use for your middle-aged and senior dog—I recommend adding this to your regular health assessments starting at the age of seven, and reviewing it every three to six months. This will give you your best chance to detect behavioral changes early so that you can discuss them with your veterinarian, who can then make sure they are or are not due to medical problems, and, if appropriate, start treatment. Recent research in AD has shown that treatment is much less effective if started when the dementia is moderate or severe, and newer therapies are being developed for use in the early stages, in hopes for greater success in slowing the cognitive decline—and this is undoubtedly true for dogs as well.

So what treatments might be available for your dog? Believe it or not, if you have a Blue Dog and have been practicing the Fab 4, you are already doing some of them! Remember "provide purpose"? You have no idea (yet) how much just that one principle can do to prevent or at least slow, cognitive decline. How about "supply structure"? The habits you have developed with your dog give him security and predictability that might be, despite your best efforts, slipping away with some of his age-related cognitive changes. When you "avoided abundance," you lessened some of the chemicals that originate in fat tissue and circulate through the body to affect the brain, and provided good nutrition to meet your dog's changing needs. And if you "dodged dental disease," you helped your dog avoid one of the risk factors that is associated with cognitive decline in humans. But if, despite these things, your dog eventually does develop some cognitive dysfunction, take heart—what you already have been doing to reduce the risk of dementia can also help slow it or partially reverse it, especially if certain supplements or medications are added.

PHYSICAL EXERCISE

Exercise is important for so many reasons. We have already covered why it is important for muscle mass, metabolic rate, weight control, and mobility, and it is one of the reasons that your dog's job has been important. Physical inactivity is *the* major risk factor for the development of AD in humans. It does so, in part, by increasing three of the other risk factors for AD—obesity, hypertension, and diabetes. But, beyond that, exercise has been actually shown to change the brain itself. It does so by:

- increasing the rate and strength of information transfer from one nerve to another
- increasing the production of Brain-Derived Neurotrophic Factor (BNDF) which essentially acts as a fertilizer of the brain's neurons, making them grow more quickly and develop stronger connections
- reducing the accumulation of reactive oxygen species
- increasing blood flow to the neurons and increasing their oxygen supply
- increasing gray matter volume
- increasing white matter volume
- increasing the size of the hippocampus—which (this is important!) improves spatial memory and increases memory consolidation—making it the gift that keeps on giving![2]

One study evaluating the impact of risk factor reduction on the development of AD found that 21 percent of the cases of AD in the United States may be attributable to physical inactivity.[3] Another study of humans with mild cognitive impairment showed that starting an exercise program caused improvements in cognitive function which were accompanied by functional and structural changes in certain brain regions as shown on MRI.[4] Aerobic exercise appears to be particularly beneficial—these are activities that stimulate and strengthen the heart and lungs, thereby improving the body's utilization of oxygen. This does not mean that older people suddenly need to take up running—the benefit to the brain appears to be induced by activities as gentle as brisk walking, swimming, dancing, and gardening. In fact, the most important factor appears to be the number of calories that are burned during the activities. Researchers at the University of California analyzed ten years of data on nearly nine hundred participants in the Cardiovascular Heart Study and found that the 25 percent most active people had substantially more gray matter than their peers, even if they had only just started to be more active in the previous few years, and that they had a 50 percent less risk of AD. Many other studies have supported the benefits to the brain of physical activity—so, whatever you do, don't stop doing something, *anything*, with your aging dog.[5]

MENTAL EXERCISE

It's important to recognize that many of the activities you do with your dog provide both physical *and* mental stimulation—for example, when you play a game like hide-and-seek, or Barn Hunt, your dog uses his nose—and, as you know, that sensory superpower takes up a lot of real estate in the canine brain. So, exercising the nose can exercise the brain! Even taking a walk with your dog gives him substantial physical and mental stimulation—every sniff your dog takes at every corner, street sign, rock, or hydrant provides his brain with a profusion of cognitively complex information. Mental inactivity is another important risk factor for the development of dementia in humans. A lot of research supports the "use it or lose it" principle of brain health—much of this has focused on the decrease in cognitive performance that occurs after people retire. Researchers suggest this is because, when retirees stop engaging in the cognitively complex tasks that came with their jobs, their brains were no longer challenged enough to maintain cognitive function.

Keep challenging your older dog, continuing to provide mentally stimulating games, activities and toys that require some complex thinking. Go to the store to buy some "food puzzles" and fill them with some extra-tasty and smelly treats—food puzzles are food-dispensing toys that require some mental and physical effort in order to obtain the reward. Keep playing games and teach new ones, especially those that require a few steps to perform—since procedural learning tends to stay sharp even as other learning declines, this will be good for your dog's confidence. Don't forget to practice your hand signals—you will need them. Also, keep visiting the Dognition.com website, and continue the games and tasks that are provided monthly. Although studies have shown that the "brain game" websites for humans don't provide the kind of cognitive challenges that truly counteract cognitive decline, the type of tasks and activities provided on the Dognition website encourage both cognitive and physical exercise which together may provide the best counterbalance to cognitive changes. One last thing—continue to practice those daily tricks—this familiar routine can be comforting for your dog, will reinforce his knowledge and confidence, and, most importantly, will make you both happy.

And happiness is good—stress is another perpetuating factor for dementia, and keeping your dog engaged and connected with you will counteract some anxiety that may occur as age-related changes to the senses, body, and mind develop. These changes can cause a sense of "distance" between the two of you—and practicing familiar routines could help him feel more connected. Also, older people and dogs have trouble handling changes that never used to bother them before, so try to keep the daily routines as consistent as possible. That being said, it is OK—in fact, good—to periodically introduce new things, such as new games, toys and the occasional new route on walks, but introduce them slowly to give your dog a chance to understand and adapt. Keep in mind that acute stress (for example, from boarding or grooming) can temporarily worsen the symptoms of cognitive dysfunction or simply induce behavioral changes that can mimic cognitive decline. These signs can improve once the acute stress is removed—in other words, don't panic, but wait to see how things are when your dog gets back to his familiar routines.

SOCIAL STIMULATION

Just in case you haven't got enough reasons to keep your dog active, here's one more—many activities and sports that provide exercise for your dog also provide opportunities for social interaction. In a large study of healthy older people, researchers found a relationship between more frequent social activity and better cognitive function. It was not clear whether improved cognition resulted from the social interactions themselves or from the increased intellectual stimulation that accompanied the social interactions. Either way, strong social ties are worth reinforcing over a lifetime, even for dogs. When your dog goes to doggie daycare or the local dog park, remember that he exercises his social muscles, too. Even if your older dog doesn't run around and play with all the other dogs as much he used to, he is still watching them interact, is reading all their social cues, and is analyzing all their scents that humans (perhaps fortunately) do not detect. Those aging neurons are getting a wake-up call every time he goes out your door—if he is left alone too much, someday they might not wake up at all.

NUTRITIONAL AND DIETARY THERAPY

Since aging, in general, is associated with progressive damage from oxygen free radicals, the brain is especially vulnerable to this type of damage since it consumes approximately 20 percent of the body's total oxygen and all those oxygen-hungry cells produce lots of free radical "waste." For much of life, the brain protects itself by cleaning up the garbage with its own waste management system, but, as time goes on, the garbage collectors become less efficient, and more and more free radicals accumulate. Free radicals are especially damaging to fat-containing cells—and, as you may remember, white matter is white because of all the fat it contains.

In terms of prevention and therapy of age-related cognitive decline, it makes sense, therefore, to focus on doing something to eliminate all those free radicals. Why, again, are free radicals bad? Remember that a stable atom has a balance between the number of positively charged components and negatively charged components. The negatively charged ones, the electrons, orbit the atom, and the positively charged ones, the protons, are in the nucleus in the center of the atom. Some atoms gain balance by acquiring electrons from other atoms, some by giving them to other atoms, and some by sharing electrons. If there are equal numbers of protons and electrons, an atom does not tend to enter into any chemical reactions. Normally, bonds don't split in a way that leaves a molecule with an odd, unpaired electron. But when weak bonds split, free radicals are formed. Free radicals are very unstable and react quickly with other compounds, trying to capture the needed electron to gain stability. Generally, free radicals attack the nearest stable molecule, "stealing" its electron. When the "attacked" molecule loses its electron, it becomes a free radical itself, beginning a chain reaction. Once the process is started, it can cascade, finally resulting in the disruption of a living cell.

A healthy, younger organism can counteract and neutralize the effects of free radicals as they are formed, but aging organisms can't always keep pace, and free radicals, along with the damage they cause, can pile up over time—unless antioxidants are consumed. Antioxidants neutralize free radicals by donating one of their own electrons, ending the electron-"stealing" chain reaction. But why don't the antioxidant nutrients become free radicals themselves when they lose an electron? That's the beauty of them—they are stable either way!

Examples of antioxidants—also known as "free-radical scavengers"—are:

- *Vitamin E*—the most abundant *fat-soluble* antioxidant in the body. Fat-soluble vitamins dissolve in fat and are stored in the fat wherever it is found in the body. It is important to know that it is difficult for the body to get rid of excess fat-soluble vitamins, so toxic levels can accumulate if too much is consumed.
- *Vitamin C*—the most abundant *water-soluble* antioxidant in the body. Water-soluble vitamins dissolve in water and act in the fluid within the cells. This type of vitamin is eliminated through the kidneys if excessive amounts are consumed. Vitamin C also helps keep Vitamin E in its active form.
- *CoEnzyme Q10* (CoQ10)—a potent antioxidant that is found in all cells, which also assists in the function of the cellular power generators, the mitochondria, and helps regulate the function of genes involved with inflammatory processes. There is some evi-

dence that CoQ10 is protective to nerve cells, and inhibits the formation of amyloid plaques. Natural levels of this substance tend to decline with age.

- *Beta-carotene*—the precursor to Vitamin A, which gives fruits and vegetables, like carrots their bright colors.
- *Alpha-lipoic acid*—an antioxidant made by the body which is found in every cell, where it helps turn glucose into energy.
- *Selenium*—a trace mineral found in many foods which is essential, in very small amounts, for many cellular processes.
- *Superoxide dismutase, catalase, glutathione peroxidase*—enzymes that defend cells against free radical damage.
- *Omega-3 fatty acids*—one of the many benefits of these essential fatty acids is to help inactivate free radicals and stabilize cell membranes.

Age-related damage to the brain, as well as other areas of the body, is due in part to poor function of the mitochondria. Logically, the goal should be to combat age-related brain changes with substances that improve mitochondrial function. The substances listed earlier help with this process, too. Another important substance that improves the function of mitochondria is *L-carnitine*—this is a substance that is made by, and found in, nearly all cells in the body. It is a favorite of bodybuilders and dieters since there is the (unfounded) belief that it helps boost energy use, improves athletic performance and promotes fat loss.

At this point, you might be wondering why I mentioned this particular group of antioxidants and mitochondrial cofactors. Well, it's because several studies in dogs have found that their addition to the diet has led to significant improvement in certain measurable parameters of cognitive function. One study followed a group of eight- to twelve-year-old dogs for a total of 2.8 years.[6] The forty-eight Beagles (housed in the lab) in the study were divided into four groups: one group received environmental enrichment (consisting of a kennel-mate, toys that were switched out once weekly, and physical exercise), one group received a custom-made diet that was supplemented with the antioxidants and mitochondrial cofactors listed previously, one received both the environmental enrichment *and* the antioxidant diet, and one (somewhat unfortunate) group received neither. Over the next 2.8 years, the dogs were tested using those convoluted tests described earlier that tested visual discrimination, landmark recognition, oddity testing, and reversal testing.

Throughout the study period, the dogs that received the antioxidant-rich diet outperformed the dogs that did not receive the enriched diet—and the differences were apparent on the landmark test only two weeks after the diet was started! Six months after the start, the enriched-diet dogs did better on the oddity tests. What is especially important about this test is that, one year after the start of the study, the group that received *both* the antioxidant diet *and* environmental enrichment were the cognitive super-stars, and this group continued to do better than all the others throughout the remainder of the study, although the diet-alone group and the environmental enrichment-alone continued to do better than the control group that received neither. The tests that the double-enriched dogs continued to do well on were those that were designed to test executive function (reversal tasks) and visual discrimination—very important abilities in day-to-day living. These findings have been supported by others, and have shown that the use of an antioxidant-rich diet led to significant improvements in social interaction, sleep patterns, disorientation, house-soiling, and activity levels.

Where, you might ask, can you get such a diet? The first one that was developed, and the one that has been researched the most, is Hill's b/d, which is available with a prescription from your veterinarian. I have prescribed this diet many times over the years and have seen cognitive improvement in several of my patients. This food incorporates a specific (and proprietary) blend of antioxidants—check with your veterinarian to see if this or another diet would be suitable for your dog's own specific medical needs.

Another diet, that uses a different strategy, is Purina One Vibrant Maturity 7+ Formula—this diet contains medium-chain triglycerides (MCTs), which are converted to substances called *ketone bodies* in the liver. Ketone bodies provide an alternate energy source for the brain—since there is a decrease in energy use by the brain as aging progresses, the provision of an additional energy source nudges the brain to keep working normally. MCTs also improve mitochondrial function, protect the fatty substances in the brain and decrease the precursors to amyloid. A study showed that this diet also improved performance of several cognitively challenging tasks.[7]

If you are tempted to supplement your dog's diet on your own, please discuss this with your vet or a veterinary nutritionist since over-supplementation can be as harmful as under-supplementation, especially if other medical problems are present. Without a degree in canine nutrition, it would be difficult to strike the right balance on your own—plus it's hard to give all the pills and capsules needed! One way to go, if you can't or don't want to feed the special diet, is to use one of these antioxidant combos:

- Cell Advance 440 (for dogs under thirty pounds) and Cell Advance 880 (for dogs over thirty pounds) by VetriScience Laboratories—it includes twenty-three antioxidants, including all of those used in the mentioned studies.
- Thorne Research Anti-Oxidant Capsules—also a good blend of the discussed antioxidants.

Or you can hit some of the antioxidant high points by giving these:

- Fruits and vegetables, especially the colorful ones that contain lots of beta-carotene like blueberries, raspberries, spinach, carrots, tomatoes and start these gradually as any new foods can cause stomach upset in dogs—but stay away from any type of grape or raisin, as they can cause kidney failure in some dogs
- Vitamin E—100 IU per day for a small dog (under 30 lb) and 400 IU per day for a large dog
- Vitamin C—50 mg per day for a small dog and 100 mg for a large dog
- CoQ10—10 mg per pound per day
- Omega-3 fatty acids—10 mg per pound per day

SUPPLEMENTS

There are several medications or supplements that may help improve the symptoms of CDS. The response is variable, and their effectiveness, or lack thereof, could be due to the degree of disease severity when they were started, or could be due to individual variations in disease expression in the brain. Discuss the potential benefits versus the potential risks with your dog's veterinarian. Ones to ask about include:

- *Selegiline (Anipryl)*—this medication, available by prescription, may act to reduce free radical production and increase levels of superoxide dismutase, the enzyme which scavenges free radicals. Improvement, if it occurs, may be seen after two to six weeks. It cannot be used with certain other drugs, such as Prozac (fluoxetine).
- *Senilife*—contains *phosphatidylserine*, which is a component of cell membranes. Older dogs that took this supplement showed improvement in tests that measured memory and learning.
- *Activait*—also contains phosphatidylserine, and tests on aged dogs that took this supplement showed a decrease in disorientation, house soiling and an improvement in social interaction.
- *Novifit*—contains S-adenosyl-L-methionine (SAMe), which increases the production of one of the body's own antioxidants, glutathione, and also helps keep cell membranes, receptors, and transmitters healthy. This one needs to be used cautiously with certain drugs, such as Prozac (fluoxetine).
- *Neutricks*—contains apoaequorin which is a protein that appears to be protective to nerves as they age.

MEDICATIONS

There are a few medications and supplements used either to slow the progression of CDS or to control some of its consequent symptoms:

- *Melatonin*—a hormone made by the pineal gland, which is a small gland in the brain which helps control sleep or wake cycles. Its synthetic form is widely available in pharmacies in the vitamin section and can be useful for dogs with night-time restlessness.
- *Prozac (fluoxetine)*—a prescription drug used for depression in humans which acts to decrease anxiety in dogs. It is often used for separation anxiety in dogs and is useful for the generalized anxiety seen in CDS.
- *Trazodone*—a prescription anti-anxiety drug which can help decrease the acute anxiety an older dog might experience in certain situations, such as boarding, grooming, or hospitalization.

- *Alprazolam (Xanax)*—a prescription medication used for the prevention or treatment of acute anxiety

This chapter provided you with a lot of information about brain aging—it may even have been somewhat overwhelming, but the reason I wanted you to have it is because I wanted to do my utmost to let you know that you have the power to shape your dog's brain destiny. Using a mash-up of two old sayings, ignorance might be bliss, but knowledge is power. Ignorance of what is going on inside your dog's brain might leave detection of the problem too late to do anything about it. If you know what to watch for—and how, and why—you can use your knowledge to protect your dog's brain and keep it as healthy as possible. You now have that—and more.

Here is a checklist to use in conjunction with your other ongoing health assessments. This is designed to help detect and categorize changes you may notice in your dog as she gets older, as some of these changes could be due to medical problems, and some could be due to early cognitive dysfunction. It can be difficult to tell the difference, especially since, as dogs age, there is a higher likelihood of both medical conditions and cognitive dysfunction—add to that the effects of stress or certain medications on the behavior of older dogs. You should show this checklist and the results to your veterinarian so that appropriate diagnostic tests and treatments, if necessary, can be started. Start using this list around the age of seven years—you are unlikely to notice changes at that age (although you might), but these early assessments, even if normal, can provide a baseline for you to make you especially aware of changes when, or if, they do occur. Remember that you are your dog's early warning system for both medical and cognitive problems, and this information will help your veterinarian sort out what is causing her symptoms.

SENIOR CHECKLIST

Part I: Physical Function Checklist

Assign these a rank of 0 (none), 1 (mild), 2 (moderate), 3 (severe)

- Has your dog gained or lost weight (or has the body condition score changed)?
- Has the appetite increased or decreased?
- Has interest in/enthusiasm for/speed of consumption of food increased or decreased?
- Increased water intake?
- Increased urine output (i.e., going outside more often to urinate)?
- Any urinary accidents? In remote places in the house or within your view?
- Any defecation in the house?
- Still signaling the need to go outside?
- After going outside, eliminates just after being back inside?
- Eliminating in crate or sleeping area?
- Any coughing?
- Weakness after exercise?
- Panting?
- Skin changes (lumps and bumps, flakiness, scabs)?
- Haircoat changes (shedding more than usual or less than usual, thinned fur, bare patches)?
- Any bad breath, red, or sore gums?
- Any difficulty chewing?
- Any shivering, shaking?
- Any weakness or incoordination?
- Any difficulty climbing stairs?
- Any stiffness? All the time or just after exercise?
- Any difficulty arising from a prone position?
- Any trouble maintaining the crouched posture needed to defecate?
- Any visual changes?
- Any changes in hearing?

Part 2: Behavior/Cognitive Function Checklist

Assign these a rank of 0 (none), 1 (mild), 2 (moderate), 3 (severe)

- Increased sleeping?
- Activity increased or decreased?
- Any wandering at night?

- Any pacing, circling, or aimless wandering?
- Any increased vocalizations (whining, barking)?
- Getting lost in house or yard?
- Going to the wrong side of the door (the hinge side)?
- Unable to navigate around or over obstacles?
- Decreased response to stimuli (touch, voice)?
- Decreased interest in being petted or touched?
- Increased need for constant contact (clingy)?
- Increased licking of people or objects?
- Still greeting you and seeming to recognize you?
- Any changes in temperament or personality?
- More irritable or aggressive?
- More anxious?
- If you have another dog, any trouble with the previously established social hierarchy?
- Staring or snapping at objects?
- Still following previously known commands?
- Still performing well-known tricks?
- Still engaging in usual play activities/games/sports?
- Seems bored or frustrated with usual play activities/games/sports?
- Able to learn new tricks?
- Able to do them again at a later time or on a different day?

21

KEEPING UP APPEARANCES

In youth we learn; in age we understand. —Marie von Ebner-Eschenbach

Let's just face it—aging isn't always pretty. But it *can* be attractive. There are positive things about aging—really there are—the wisdom that comes from experience, the ease that comes from familiarity, the peace that comes from confidence. However, there are indeed some physical trappings that inevitably accompany age. Your bouncy, shiny puppy will undoubtedly change a lot over the years, and, then again, so will you. But how you look at your dog, and, maybe at yourself, should not. You won't know this unless you've aged a bit yourself, but what you see when you look in the mirror, or when you picture yourself in your mind's eye, will have more to do with how your own body image used to be when it was first formed in early adulthood and less to do with the reality that other people see when they look at you. I am always a little surprised when I see a photo of myself and think "Who *is* that older woman—my mother?" Sure, in my fifties, I have some wrinkles, some (tastefully concealed) gray hair, some crackly joints—but I really don't *feel* any different than I did when I was in my twenties. My attitude toward myself, my sense of self, my *essence* hasn't aged—whatever it is that makes me *me*, hasn't changed along with my body. It will be the same for you—and it will be the same for your dog. Your dog has no real sense of the time that has passed since you first brought her home, and deals with life and aging as it unfolds just as she always has—simply doing what she does without thinking about it—or looking in the mirror. You, however, might note the gray muzzle, the cloudy-appearing eyes, the hitch in her get-along—and might regard those changes with a measure of sadness—maybe even pity.

Don't do that! Don't, whatever you do, fall into the trap of *ageism*—which is defined as the "tendency to regard older persons as debilitated, unworthy of attention, or unsuitable for employment." In our youth-oriented society, there is a predisposition to, at best, patronize older people, and, at worst, denigrate them. For my part, I hate it when someone younger that I, whom I've never met before calls me "dear" or "sweetheart"—that person knows nothing about me, and I immediately feel as if I have been put in a box of limited expectations. I am just as full of possibilities and abilities as I ever was—and my age actually has little relevance to how I live my life. What has relevance is the butterfly effect of the millions of small decisions I have made, the minute influences that I have had on other people and the influences they have had on me, and the continual course corrections I have made in my route through life. I live, and learn, and then I live and learn some more. In a way, I regard my life up to this point as a source of knowledge—about life, about people, about myself—and I plan to use that knowledge to safely navigate the future, since the past and the present are the only way to actually *get* to the future. That is the way you should think about your dog, no matter what age she is.

Over the years, you've had the opportunity to truly understand your dog, inside and out, and have used that knowledge to confidently guide her to her future. You know by now what she is capable of—physically, mentally—and you need to keep pushing the edges of her envelope. Although you may have to make some accommodation for some age-related changes, you can still focus on her abilities instead of her disabilities. If you put *her* in a box of limited expectations, she'll just be *old*.

"Age-proofing" is really a matter of attitude—well, actually, only one attitude—*yours*. Your dog will truly be age-proofed if you look past the chronology and cosmetics that indicate her age and see all the things that have made her *her* throughout her life. Whatever sparked her soul when she came into your life will still be glowing inside her no matter what the clock says. And if you keep looking for that spark, while continuing to feed it and cherish it, your dog will never be old. After all, according to the all-time expert on age-proofing: "All you need is a little faith, trust, and pixie dust" —Peter Pan.

22

TAKING STOCK

Somewhere between the bottom of the climb and the summit is the
answer to the mystery why we climb. —Greg Child

So far in this book, we have been focusing on all the things that you can
do to extend your dog's healthspan—the period during life free of serious illness and disability—which may, in turn, help extend your dog's
lifespan—the period between birth and death. Have you noticed the
presence of the word "span" within each of those two words? The
definition of the word span is: "an extent, stretch, reach, or spread
between two limits." This, of course, implies that, no matter what we do
in life, there is a limit to it. In the same way, the fact that we, and our
dogs, are alive suggests that we, and they, will someday not be. Despite
the inevitability of an end, at some point, to the time you and your dog
have together, each stage of your dog's life that you have experienced
together will have been an opportunity for learning, growth, wisdom—
and love.

As you and your dog go through your long life's trek together, emphasize, in your mind, the journey, not the end—but at the same time,
don't fear the end. In death, you actually discover the life that has
ended, and realize the impact that particular life has had on you. Despite the grief and sadness that you will inevitably feel, you will continue to remember the love, the comfort, the laughs—and the purpose to
your own life that your dog gave you. Your dog's life enriched yours
during the time that life persisted, and will do so after death as well.

Pull out your time capsule from time to time as your dog gets older, and also after he is gone—what you wrote down all those years ago will remind you what made that individual dog so special then, and what still makes him so special now. It will help you remember the ways he enhanced your life, and the ways in which he enhanced yours. Reminding yourself of all the elements that are unique only to you and your dog's relationship will help you maintain and promote them as the years go on, and will help you realize when some of them are fading. This will help you recognize the time toward the end of life when the spark that made that dog *your dog* has dimmed, and will help you come to terms with the limit to his life. Later, reviewing what you wrote down about your dog so long ago will give you some comfort, some reassurance that your lives together were well lived, and that the climb to the top was worth the effort. It's always worth the effort.

As you reach the summit of your dog's life, you will need help along the way. If, despite all you have done to keep your dog's arthritic limbs comfortable, he develops pain—there are always more ways to help. If despite all you have done, your dog develops kidney disease, or cancer, or becomes unable to get outside and then soils himself—there are always more ways to help.

The field of animal hospice has expanded in recent years, and exists to support and care for dogs just like yours and for people just like you. Hospice veterinarians come to your home to alleviate your dog's pain, administer fluids and medications, and help with hygiene—their emphasis is to continue to allow patients to live life as fully as possible and as comfortably as possible even though the end of life is near, whether through natural death or euthanasia. Your own veterinarian may provide some of these services and may advise you on how to care for your dog, but not all veterinarians are able to help in this way.

Sometimes, veterinarians adopt an "either/or" mentality to end-of-life care—a veterinarian may give a patient a diagnosis (such as cancer), and gives the owner the choice of *either* doing something the owner doesn't feel comfortable with (such as chemotherapy) *or* putting the dog to sleep right then. Sometimes, a veterinarian may say there is nothing else to do for your aged dog, and say that the only option is euthanasia.

There are always other choices, and you, if faced with this type of situation, need to know it is OK to explore them. Discuss this with your veterinarian and also go to the International Association of Animal Hospice and Palliative Care (iaahpc.org) to check their directory for hospice providers in your area. This website also has helpful information about hospice and palliative care for animals, as well as many links that may become useful as time goes on.

At some point, you will need to ask the question that nobody wants to ask—"Is it time?" Most dog owners wish they would never have to make a decision to end their dog's life, and would choose a natural death for their dog—but, often, a natural death only occurs after a period of discomfort or distress. There is nothing wrong with waiting for death to occur, as long as pain is eased and suffering is prevented—but this is difficult to watch and can lead to so much more sorrow than even the death itself would cause. Many people wish to allow their dogs to die before they have suffered, and, that way, despite the anguish that the people experience in making the decision, at least their dogs go through less distress overall. It is, however, very difficult to know just when it *is* time.

When my clients ask me how they will know when to make the decision to euthanize their dog, I tell them that the decision is unique to each situation, and that there is not one clear answer. I first ask them to think about what it is that makes their dog the special individual he is— what little habits, what little quirks of personality, what specific likes and dislikes he has—and to ask themselves if those things are still there. I then ask if they think their dog is in any pain, that has been unable to be alleviated by medications. I also ask them if he is having difficulty in acquiring food, water, and air, which are, obviously, needed for life— and to consider how distressing it might be for their dog to know he needs these things, but is unable to get them. After all, our brains are programmed to make us do whatever we can to sustain life, and it is very stressful when we also know we can't do them. I tell people that this is a different kind of pain, but is pain nonetheless. I ask if their dog's bad days outnumber his good days—but first I ask them to define what a good day is for their dog, and what a bad day is. Last, I ask them to look into their dog's eyes and see if he is still looking back. This is one thing that can't be described, but everybody seems to know what it means.

In addition, I will often tell my clients the story of the time when my husband and I were faced with this decision for our dog, Ryder, the arthritic, elderly, rescued Golden Retriever I mentioned earlier. At about the age of fifteen, Ryder began to be incontinent of urine. After a urinalysis and X-rays didn't reveal the source of the problem, an abdominal ultrasound did—an inoperable bladder tumor. At the time of diagnosis, Ryder was as happy, social, and ball-crazy as ever. He didn't know he had cancer—we did, and we knew that we would eventually have to make a decision—but, at first, the only day-to-day problem we had was the incontinence. So we put a diaper on him, and decided on this plan: we decided that when Ryder's bad days outnumbered his good days, we would talk to each other about putting him to sleep.

This was fine, but a little too vague—so we defined what a good day was for Ryder. A good day for Ryder was to be interested in, and affectionate toward, his family, to display his usual gusto for food, and to love his tennis balls above almost all else. A bad day for Ryder was the lack of one or all of those things. We also went a little further—we decided that, in the absence of overt pain, we would allow him to have three consecutive bad days, and then, we would talk and discuss whether it was time. This plan worked out well for us—and for Ryder. Over the next twelve months, Ryder remained his goofy, happy self—but eventually he did start to have a bad day here and a bad day there. Then there might be two in a row—and, again, he would bounce back. But almost exactly one year after diagnosis, he did have three bad days—not too bad, but they did satisfy the criteria we had set forth—and we knew exactly what we should do. The burden of a very emotional, subjective decision had been lifted off by the more objective guidelines we had made for ourselves, and that kept us from constantly asking ourselves throughout the year whether it was "time." We knew exactly what to do, and we could then relax to cherish the remaining time we had left, before I eased him to sleep on our patio, in the sunshine, with my husband holding his paw, while Ryder watched the birds and laid his head on his collection of worn tennis balls.

The decision you make for your own dog will be as unique as your life together, and your relationship throughout it. There are no right or wrong decisions—only the one that is right for you. If you do seek euthanasia for your dog, you may or may not wish to be present—again, there is no right or wrong way. But please be aware that it is a painless process—at least to the body—although not to our hearts. The medications that are used are all anesthesia drugs, and most veterinarians first use a sedative, and then follow that with a stronger version of the first drug that slows down the heart and breathing until it eventually stops. Keep in mind that anesthesia was invented for good reason—to relieve pain, to alleviate stress, and to induce a sense of well-being and euphoria. This is, after all, why so many people are addicted to these drugs—they will actually make your dog feel quite good. I believe that dogs are a "here and now" species—they know what they know at the time that they know it, feel what they feel at the time that they feel it, and don't reflect upon it much.

As the medications used for euthanasia are going in, pain is eased, stress is reduced, and dogs feel that change and know that they feel better. Even though they will soon fall asleep, they don't know that they will not be waking up—they only know that they feel better, and, to them, it is not so different from falling asleep at home, surrounded by their family and infused with love and comfort—just like they have done thousands of times before. Humans know the difference, and might have doubt, or guilt, or be filled with "what ifs"—but this is the moment to think like a dog—perhaps the most caninomorphic moment of all. When this moment comes for your dog, realize that, in the few seconds before he falls asleep, he is pain-free, and has no other focus at that time except you and your love. Think like your dog at that time, and just pour love and comfort into each other. It's not a bad last thought to give him—or yourself.

23

AND THEN . . . ?

When one door of happiness closes, another opens; but often we look
so long at the closed door that we do not see the one that has been
opened for us. —Helen Keller

Despite all our preparation for the death of Ryder, we couldn't really
"grief-proof" ourselves once it happened. To make matters worse, we
had lost our other Golden Retriever, Ezra, just three weeks before, due
to a quick-growing and painful tumor. My husband, in particular, was
devastated, and he was also concerned about the impact these two
deaths would have on our daughters. He soon suggested that we look
for another dog to rescue—"for the girls"—but I knew it was really for
him. We checked the Central Indiana Golden Retriever Rescue website—and, low and behold, five three-week-old Golden Retriever puppies had been rescued, along with their mother! We hadn't been planning on a puppy—but what better way is there to bring a smile to
someone's face? We went to check them out and planned to choose
one—and, of course, came home with two! That, by the way, is the story
of Fiona and Shrek.

What was strange about this was that Shrek turned out to be practically a clone of Ryder—his personality was the same, his mobility (unfortunately for him) was about the same as an old dog, and he was, after
his stem cell treatment, every bit as goofy and ball-crazy. You might not
think that is not all that surprising—after all, they were the same
breed—but so was Fiona, and she didn't act anything like Ryder—oddly
enough, she was more like Ezra. For us, Shrek and Fiona were not, and

never could be, a replacement for Ryder and Ezra—they were more like tributes to them. We will never have another Ryder, or another Ezra, and our lives with Fiona and Shrek have been vastly different than our lives with their predecessors. In part, it is because we have changed—my husband and I are at a different stage of life now than we were then, and we probably have different expectations of our dogs than we did before. Our dogs fill different roles in our empty-nest lives now and they will continue to evolve as we evolve. Despite that, when a smiling Shrek brings a soggy tennis ball for me to throw, or a sweet Fiona hands me her paw to hold, I see a glimmer of Ryder in him and a glimmer of Ezra in her—and I remember the gifts those two gave us all those years ago. Someday, when Fiona and Shrek are gone, some other dog, with a turn of the head, or a prick of the ear, will remind us of them, and those before them—and the cycle will continue until we no longer have life ourselves.

For us, we found life after death. For you, things may be different. There is no right way or wrong way to recover from the loss of a life companion. But recover you will. You may want to get another dog right away to assuage your pain and plug up the hole left in your life, or you may not want another one for a while—or ever. Either way, you will be OK. One word of advice, however—be sure to keep the spark of your dog alive in your mind as time goes on. It will comfort you and sustain you as the moment of loss fades and the memories of the long, wonderful life that preceded it grow stronger. Plus you never know—you might see that spark in someone else's eyes someday. That is, if you look . . .

NOTES

3. THE INNER GAME OF DOG

1. Nathan B. Sutter et al., "A Single IGF1 Allele Is a Major Determinant of Small Size in Dogs," *Science* 316, no. 5821 (2007): 112–15.

2. Adam R. Boyko et al., "A Simple Genetic Architecture Underlies Morphological Variation in Dogs," *PLoS Biology* 8, no. 8 (2010): 112–15.

3. David Grimm, "Dogs May Have Been Domesticated More than Once," *Science* 3, no. 352(6290) (June 2016): 1153–54.

4. Brian Hare and Vanessa Woods, *The Genius of Dogs: How Dogs Are Smarter than You Think* (New York: Dutton, 2013), 119–21.

5. Heidi G. Parker, "Genomic Analyses of Modern Dog Breeds," *Mammalian Genome* 23, no. 1–2 (2012): 19–27.

6. Heidi G. Parker et al., "Breed Relationships Facilitate Fine-Mapping Studies: A 7.8-kb Deletion Cosegregates with Collie Eye Anomaly across Multiple Dog Breeds," *Genome Research* 17, no. 11 (2007): 1562–71.

7. Thomas J. Bouchard Jr. and John C. Loehlin, "Genes, Evolution and Personality," *Behavioral Genetics* no. 3 (May 31, 2001): 243–73.

8. Kenth Svartberg and Bjorn Forkman, "Personality Traits in the Domestic Dog (*Canis familiaris*)," *Applied Animal Behavior Science* 79, no. 2 (October 20, 2002): 133–55.

4. THE INNER GAME OF *YOUR* DOG

1. Amanda C. Jones, "Development and Validation of a Dog Personality Questionnaire." (PhD diss., University of Texas, Austin, 2009); Samuel D. Gos-

ling, Virginia S. Y. Kwan, and Oliver P. John, "A Dog's Got Personality: A Cross-Species Comparative Approach to Personality Judgments in Dogs and Humans," *Journal of Personality and Social Psychology* 85, no. 6 (2003): 1161–69.

2. Borbála Turcsán et al., "Birds of a Feather Flock Together? Perceived Personality Matching in Owner-Dog Dyads," *Applied Animal Behaviour Science* 140, no. 3 (2012): 154–60.

3. Anthony L. Podberscek and James A. Serpell, "Aggressive Behaviour in English Cocker Spaniels and the Personality of Their Owners," *Veterinary Record* 141, no. 3 (1997): 73–76.

4. Valerie O'Farrell, "Owner Attitudes and Dog Behaviour Problems," *Applied Animal Behaviour Science* 52, no. 3 (1997): 205–13.

6. GETTING TO KNOW *ALL* ABOUT YOU

1. Christine Nießner et al., "Cryptochrome 1 in Retinal Cone Photoreceptors Suggests a Novel Functional Role in Mammals," *Scientific Reports* 6 (2016): 21848.

7. THE LAUDATORY AUDITORY

1. Attila Andics, Márta Gácsi, Tamás Faragó, Anna Kis, and Ádám Miklósi, "Voice-Sensitive Regions in the Dog and Human Brain Are Revealed by Comparative FMRI," *Current Biology* 24, no. 5 (2014): 574–78.

2. M. Fukuzawa, D. S. Mills, and J. J. Cooper, "The Effect of Human Command Phonetic Characteristics on Auditory Cognition in Dogs (Canis Familiaris)," *Journal of Comparative Psychology* 119, no. 1 (2005): 117–20.

3. Juliane Kaminski, Josep Call, and Julia Fischer, "Word Learning in a Domestic Dog: Evidence for 'Fast Mapping,'" *Science* 304, no. 5677 (2004): 1682–83.

10. BLUE DOGS

1. Dan Buettner, *The Blue Zones: Lessons for Living Longer from the People Who've Lived the Longest* (Washington, DC: National Geographic Society, 2008).

11. PROVIDE PURPOSE

1. Laughlin Stewart et al., "Citizen Science as a New Tool in Dog Cognition Research," *PLoS ONE* 10, no. 9 (2015). doi:10.1371/journal.pone.0135176.

13. PRACTICE PREVENTION

1. Jennifer E. Rawlinson et al., "Association of Periodontal Disease with Systemic Health Indices in Dogs and the Systemic Response to Treatment of Periodontal Disease," *Journal of the American Veterinary Medical Association* 238, no. 5 (2011): 601–9.

2. H. E. Kortegaard, T. Eriksen, and V. Baelum, "Periodontal Disease in Research Beagle Dogs—An Epidemiological Study," *Journal of Small Animal Practice* 49, no. 12 (2008): 610–16.

14. CH-CH-CH-CHANGES . . . TRENDS TO WATCH FOR IN MIDDLE AGE AND BEYOND

1. Jan Bellows et al., "Defining Healthy Aging in Older Dogs and Differentiating Healthy Aging from Disease," *Journal of the American Veterinary Medical Association* 246, no. 1 (2015): 77–89.

15. BEWARE THE CREEP

1. Anna Maria Mello, Giulia Paroni, Julia Daragjati, and Alberto Pilotto, "Gastrointestinal Microbiota and Their Contribution to Healthy Aging," *Digestive Diseases* 34, no. 3 (2016): 194–201.

16. SHIFTING SENSES

1. D. L. Williams, M. F. Heath, and C. Wallis, "Prevalence of Canine Cataract: Preliminary Results of a Cross-Sectional Study," *Veterinary Ophthalmology* 7.1 (2004): 29–35.

2. Silvan R. Urfer, Kimberly Greer, and Norman S. Wolf, "Age-Related Cataract in Dogs: A Biomarker for Life Span and Its Relation to Body Size," *Age* 33, no. 3 (2010): 451–60.

3. S. G. Rosolen et al., "The Effect of Aging on the Retinal Function in Two Selected Breeds of Dogs," *Investigative Ophthalmology and Visual Sciences* 51, no. 13 (2005): 5577.

17. TURN UP THE VOLUME

1. G. Ter Haar, A. J. Venker-van Haagen, W. E. Van Den Brom, F. J. Van Sluijs, and G. F. Smoorenburg, "Effects of Aging on Brainstem Responses to Toneburst Auditory Stimuli: A Cross-Sectional and Longitudinal Study in Dogs," *Journal of Veterinary Internal Medicine* 22, no. 4 (2008): 937–45.

2. Tima Le and Elizabeth M. Keithley, "Effects of Antioxidants on the Aging Inner Ear," *Hearing Research* 226, no. 1 (2007): 194–202; Akinori Shimada, Manami Ebisu, Takehito Morita, Takashi Takeuchi, and Takashi Umemura, "Age-Related Changes in the Cochlea and Cochlear Nuclei of Dogs," *Journal of Veterinary Medical Science* 60, no. 1 (1998): 41–48.

3. Carly L. Mason, Susan Paterson, and Peter J. Cripps, "Use of a Hearing Loss Grading System and an Owner-Based Hearing Questionnaire to Assess Hearing Loss in Pet Dogs with Chronic Otitis Externa or Otitis Media," *Veterinary Dermatology* 24, no. 5 (2013): 512–e121.

4. Peter Scheifele, Doug Martin, John Greer Clark, Debra Kemper, and Jennifer Wells, "Effect of Kennel Noise on Hearing in Dogs," *American Journal of Veterinary Research* 73, no. 4 (2012): 482–89.

18. DIMINISHING RETURNS

1. T. Hirai et al., "Age-related Changes in the Olfactory System of Dogs," *Neuropathology and Applied Neurobiology* 22, no. 6 (1996): 531–39.

2. J. Armando Villamil et al., "Identification of the Most Common Cutaneous Neoplasms in Dogs and Evaluation of Breed and Age Distributions for Selected Neoplasms," *Journal of the American Veterinary Medical Association* 239, no. 7 (2011): 960–65.

19. STICKY WICKETS

1. Caiqiong Hu et al., "Acupuncture for Pain Management in Cancer: A Systematic Review and Meta-Analysis," *Evidence-Based Complementary and Alternative Medicine* 2016 (2016): 1–13.

2. James K. Roush et al., "Evaluation of the Effects of Dietary Supplementation with Fish Oil Omega-3 Fatty Acids on Weight Bearing in Dogs with Osteoarthritis," *Journal of the American Veterinary Medical Association* 236, no. 1 (2010): 67–73.

3. Dale A. Fritsch et al., "A Multicenter Study of the Effect of Dietary Supplementation with Fish Oil Omega-3 Fatty Acids on Carprofen Dosage in Dogs with Osteoarthritis," *Journal of the American Veterinary Medical Association* 236, no. 5 (2010): 535–39; Anna Hielm-Björkman et al., "An Un-commissioned Randomized, Placebo-Controlled Double-Blind Study to Test the Effect of Deep Sea Fish Oil as a Pain Reliever for Dogs Suffering from Canine OA," *BMC Veterinary Research* 8, no. 1 (2012): 157. 10.1186/1746-6148-8 -157.

4. James K. Roush et al., "Multicenter Veterinary Practice Assessment of the Effects of Omega-3 Fatty Acids on Osteoarthritis in Dogs," *Journal of the American Veterinary Medical Association* 236, no. 1 (2010): 59–66.

5. L. L. Black et al., "Effect of Adipose-Derived Mesenchymal Stem and Regenerative Cells on Lameness in Dogs with Chronic Osteoarthritis of the Coxofemoral Joints: A Randomized, Double-Blinded, Multicenter, Controlled Trial," *Veterinary Therapy* 8, no. 4 (2007): 272–84.

6. Jose M. Vilar et al., "Assessment of the Effect of Intraarticular Injection of Autologous Adipose-Derived Mesenchymal Stem Cells in Osteoarthritic Dogs Using a Double Blinded Force Platform Analysis," *BMC Veterinary Research* 10, no. 1 (2014): 143. doi:10.1186/1746-6148-10-143.

20. FUZZY LOGIC

1. Christina T. Siwak-Tapp et al., "Neurogenesis Decreases with Age in the Canine Hippocampus and Correlates with Cognitive Function," *Neurobiology of Learning and Memory* 88, no. 2 (2007): 249–59.

2. K. I. Erickson et al., "Exercise Training Increases Size of Hippocampus and Improves Memory," *Proceedings of the National Academy of Sciences* 108, no. 7 (2011): 3017–22; Shikha Snigdha, Christina De Rivera, Norton W. Milgram, and Carl W. Cotman, "Exercise Enhances Memory Consolidation in the Aging Brain," *Frontiers in Aging Neuroscience* 6 (2014).

3. Deborah E. Barnes and Kristine Yaffe, "The Projected Effect of Risk Factor Reduction on Alzheimer's Disease Prevalence," *The Lancet Neurology* 10, no. 9 (2011): 819–28.

4. Pei Huang, Rong Fang, Bin-Yin Li, and Sheng-Di Chen, "Exercise-Related Changes of Networks in Aging and Mild Cognitive Impairment Brain," *Frontiers in Aging Neuroscience* 8 (2016).

5. Cyrus A. Raji et al., "Longitudinal Relationships between Caloric Expenditure and Gray Matter in the Cardiovascular Health Study," *Journal of Alzheimer's Disease* 52, no. 2 (2016): 719–29.

6. N. W. Milgram et al., "Learning Ability in Aged Beagle Dogs Is Preserved by Behavioral Enrichment and Dietary Fortification: A Two-Year Longitudinal Study," *Neurobiology of Aging* 26, no. 1 (2005): 77–90.

7. Yuanlong Pan et al., "Dietary Supplementation with Medium-Chain TAG Has Long-Lasting Cognition-Enhancing Effects in Aged Dogs," *British Journal of Nutrition* 103, no. 12 (2010): 1746–54.

INDEX

Note: Page numbers in *italics* refer to images such as photographs, diagrams, and charts.

ABOUT THE AUTHOR

Elizabeth U. Murphy, DVM, is a small-animal veterinarian and former physician assistant who has practiced for the past nineteen years at the innovative and progressive Broad Ripple Animal Clinic in Indianapolis, Indiana. Murphy has been a regular contributor to NPR's *Sound Medicine* radio show and podcast where she explores the many parallels between human and veterinary medicine. Murphy provides information to pet owners about the ways to help their dogs age gracefully and age well on her website and blog: howtoageproofyourdog.com. Murphy may also be followed on Twitter (@howtoageproofyourdog) as well as Facebook (https://www.facebook.com/pages/How-To-Age-Proof-Your-Dog). Murphy is a popular local speaker and has contributed to *Veterinary Trends* magazine. She is also an animal portraitist, and her artwork may be viewed on her website at: artisticbuzz.com.